The Mindbody Cleanse

by Ronly Blau and Adrian Nowland

This book is not intended to diagnose, treat or prescribe any medical condition. The information contained in this book is not intended to replace your own inner guidance or consultation with your healthcare professional.

May this book serve you in your journey to realizing your best self. We wish you health, happiness and deep peace.

ISBN 978-0-692-64677-9

Library of Congress Control Number: 2016936180

Cover photos (front and back) by Nealy Blau
Cover design by Jenna Riggs Collaborative

Deep gratitude for your generous help and support:
Nealy Blau, Katie Konrad, Joseph Panzetta, Kathryn True,
Simon Watson, Rich and Mary Watson

And, to all our teachers, with a deep bow to:
Heather Martin, Kathleen Hunt, John Douillard, Dr. Vasant Lad, Cynthia Copple, Dr.
Sarita Shrestha, Dr. Robert Svoboda, Sarah Powers, Anne Cushman, Melanie Farmer,
Niika Quistgard, David Crow and Dr. Jayarajan Kodikannath

Contents

*"Like with any journey, it's not what you carry,
but what you leave behind."*

—Robyn Davidson, Tracks

Foreword

I first met Ronly Blau when she enrolled at Mount Madonna Institute, where I was co-founder and Dean. She was one of our best students, so full of the joy of learning. I observed her growing in knowledge, wisdom and compassion month by month, year by year. She had so many questions and was determined to find the answers.

In 1982 Dr. R.P. Trivedi gave me the mission to "bring Ayurveda to the West." Although it seemed clear to me that Ayurveda was needed in America to help people stay healthy and heal on the physical, mental, emotional and spiritual level, it appeared that very few people understood or cared about the connection between diet, lifestyle, genetic inheritance, stress and health. Still, there was nobody else to do it so I continued to practice and teach Ayurveda and with like-minded individuals create organizations such as the National Ayurvedic Medical Association (which we established in 2000).

Now the western scientific and medical world is "discovering" truths known 5,000 years ago by Ayurveda, such as the Ayurvedic body/mind "type", similar to the western "genotype." The impact of emotions, stress, diet and exercise on health and disease, which ancient Ayurveda specifically described, is finally being "proven" by western science.

Ronly and Adrian are carrying this mission to the next step in The Mindbody Cleanse. It is my wish that many people read and practice what they are teaching.

In The Mindbody Cleanse, the authors' mastery of Ayurvedic knowledge is evident. They clearly explain classical Pancha Karma and have created a 14 day cleanse that will benefit just about everyone. In over 25 years of offering Pancha Karma at my clinic, I have seen many positive results and am so glad they are bringing this understanding to more people.

Their personal results from Ayurvedic cleansing are impressive. They exemplify the reason we founded Mount Madonna Institute College of Ayurveda—to train practitioners to heal the world that was in such need of it. It still is!

- Cynthia Copple

INTRODUCTION

The mind and body together act as the lens from which we know and experience all phenomena. Through each of the senses, thoughts and emotions, we absorb the myriad of wonders life has to offer. In effect, the quality, efficiency and clarity of our living experience is directly influenced by the quality, efficiency and clarity of the mind and body. Cleaning the lens will help us see clearly! And, regular cleansing is integral to maintaining health and longevity in the mindbody vehicle.

Cleansing is a Deeply Healing Experience

This 14-day cleanse from Ayurveda is a deep and holistic detoxification process that has long-lasting effects. The methods in this book are based on traditional *panchakarma* cleansing therapies from ancient Ayurvedic medicine and adapted for home use. Unlike many cleansing fads, it has endured the test of time and goes deeper than a temporary digestive re-haul. While following the methods outlined in this book, you will likely experience increased energy and mental clarity, a lighter body, decreased allergies, decreased body pain and improved digestion. However, this cleanse takes you even further. It improves the physiological efficiency of the body through the regulation of blood sugar, healing and strengthening the digestive system, and rejuvenating our natural detoxification pathways. And still, the more profound result of cleansing the Ayurvedic way lies in the transformational relationship you develop with food, habitual thought patterns and, ultimately, yourself.

In the Mindbody Cleanse, we emphasize three branches: 1) Diet and Herbs, 2) Stress Management and 3) Self-care.

Through the diet and herbal protocol, you clear out the gunk (*ama*) that has been building up in the body's numerous channels. Consequently, the inherent life force (*prana*) can flow through the body with renewed freedom and intelligence.

Through the stress management branch, you learn to manage the tricky mind that tends to struggle with life as it strives to make it into a desirable form. With the practice of yoga, pranayama and meditation, the mind becomes gathered - focused in the moment. In this state, there is a chance for your innate wisdom to guide you and to surrender to the flow of life.

The self-care branch provides the opportunity to make life-altering changes through simple, nurturing habits. You slow down enough to notice your life experience: attitudes and attachments around food, emotional patterns that arise unbidden from the same old stories, moments of your own inner stillness. In these moments, you have a choice. You can choose to live more skillfully, making healthy choices with food and lifestyle.

Our Relationship to Food

In the fast pace of life, food is used for many reasons, not just to fuel the body. The simple and nutritious recipes in this cleanse highlight food as a source of nourishment, a shift from typical patterns. This approach will clear the space for you to ask yourself: what am I distracting myself from by eating? Do I reach for food when I am feeling bored, angry, scared, lazy, sad, anxious, nervous? What cravings do I have on a daily basis that I don't recognize because I quickly satisfy it with something? What do these cravings mean?

This awareness can break the cycle of food addiction. The cleanse diet is simple and easy. It is utilized long enough to notice the negative effects that refined sugar, caffeine and junk food have on your body, brain and life. These substances create a physiological dependency. Research shows that white sugar is more addictive than cocaine. With this knowledge, it is no wonder sugar has silently slipped into nearly every packaged food on the grocery store shelves. We're addicted!

By stripping down the number of foods you are eating for two weeks, the slate is primed for new, positive habits to take hold. At the end of this book there is an entire section devoted to eating — when you're not cleansing — to maintain daily detoxification and ultimate vitality.

The Big Picture
This cleanse is an opportunity to open your consciousness and welcome your highest self into existence. When you slow down and tune in, you begin to understand the subtle changes that food, breath work, yoga and meditation can make on your mind and body. These can affect your mood, body temperature, appearance, state of mind, health, energy and relationships. Ayurveda has been teaching this for thousands of years. With this increased

awareness, you will have the opportunity to break old patterns that are no longer serving you and to welcome in new ways of being that are more skillful.

The mechanism for true transformation is this awareness. As one Ayurvedic teacher put it, "awareness is guru." It is one thing to cleanse the mindbody every year. But, if you are not taking steps to transform, then most likely the patterns that led to the toxic buildup in the first place will resurface and you will be back to the same place the following year. When you take notice and accurately see your relationship to food and lifestyle, the cause and effect of your life choices becomes clear. With this clarity, wisdom has a chance to direct your choices and the old unhealthy habitual patterns begin to atrophy and fall away from disuse.

Cleansing the Mind
The body is made up of thousands of channels, from the more obvious like the gastrointestinal tract, to the subtle channels within each cell membrane. It is through these channels that the body is nourished and through them that the body detoxifies. It is like any plumbing issue — once the obstructions are removed from the pipes, the flow will return. In the body, good flow through the channels means you can efficiently absorb energy and information. You are well nourished, able to repair problematic areas and can properly eliminate wastes.

In Ayurveda, the mind is considered another channel. It is the mind's ability to function well that sows the seeds for health. On a practical level, you are able to see what is best for yourself and to act upon those instincts. In Ayurveda, when the mind is peaceful, fulfilled, clear and stable, it is referred to as *sattvic*.

The sense organs are the openings to the mind channel. Sense organs (eyes, nose, mouth, skin and ears) are what connect the outer world with inner experience. When you begin to clear the toxins (ama) out of the body during cleansing, the sense organs become well-tuned and sharp. Consequently, you are able to perceive the world with less distortion from mind and body, cultivating a sattvic state. And it is the sattvic mind that provides the window into universal consciousness and true nature. With clear knowing, you can observe what is happening in the moment. This is the aware quality that is the portal to transformation and healing.

Blessings on Your Journey

The pages ahead will take you on a healing inner journey. Physically and emotionally many wonderful things may happen to you, but the greatest potential in this cleanse lies in that potent combination of a clear body and mind which is conducive to living with more awareness. When the body and mind are clear and peaceful, you are connected to your innate wisdom and the universal intelligence throughout the cosmos.

We encourage you to enter this sacred journey with an open mind, a full heart and a sense of discovery. Be wildly curious about who you are, what is important to you and where you want to go. Most importantly, love yourself. Be kind to yourself. Slow down, tune in and unearth what has been waiting there.

How to Use This Book

We suggest reading the entire book before beginning your cleanse — or at least visiting each section so you have a sense of the entire scope of this cleanse before starting your program. Having some background about Ayurveda — where this cleanse comes from — as well as your constitution and the protocol may affect the way you want to individualize your cleanse. For instance, if you notice after taking the Dosha (constitution) Quiz that you have a lot of vata (air and space) tendencies, you may want to prioritize scheduling a professional abhyanga massage. If you are already an Ayurvedaphile or want to jump right into the cleanse, you can certainly start on Chapter 5 and read the other sections at your leisure.

Studying the map for this journey will allow you to surrender to the process with understanding and trust. These qualities are beneficial because when we have knowledge and trust, we can relax. When we relax, our bodies soften. The channels of the body, no longer constricted, can open and facilitate the release of toxins and stored emotions. This encourages a deeper detoxification than what diet alone can do. Once you have looked through the book, you can follow the protocol in the order it is presented. Do check out the section on herbs in Chapter 7, The Preparation Phase, so you can have any herbal supplements on-hand before starting your cleanse. We also recommend taking the shopping list found at the beginning of the Recipe section to the store and getting all food supplies beforehand.

Throughout the book we use Sanskrit terms, for which we provide a definition. If these are distracting, skip over them; if they are helpful or interesting, absorb as much as you can. Sometimes we use the Sanskrit term over and over again (such as ama — toxins) and you will find that you come to understand their meaning without having to read the translation.

Contraindications

This method of cleansing is not recommended under the following conditions: pregnancy, nursing, severe weakness, melanoma, lymphosarcoma, cancer of the lungs or testicles, HIV or AIDS, untreated hypertension, heart disease or any active infectious disease. If you have any underlying condition or health concerns, it is best to do this cleanse in consultation with your physician and an Ayurvedic practitioner.

For women:
It is best to plan the purification week outside the time of menses. However, if menses should occur during this time, the cleanse can be moderated. See the Troubleshooting section on page 115 - 117.

Our Stories

Ronly's Story

I often say that before I went to study Ayurveda at the Mount Madonna Institute, I went to a much tougher College — that of my own body. I became aware of Ayurveda through my own health struggles and subsequent healing process. I had severe chronic sinusitis for at least eight years, and had gone from being a professional dancer, often rehearsing five hours per day, to a barely-able-to-get-out-of-bed mom of two babes living in survival mode. During that time I saw three MDs, four NDs, a craniosacral practitioner, an acupuncturist, psychotherapist, shamanic healer and, lastly, an Ayurvedic practitioner. After I began working within the Ayurvedic model, I finally started to show signs of healing. This is not to imply that the other modalities did not help or have value, only that it took the holistic nature of Ayurveda to get to the root cause of the imbalance. Ayurveda addressed the many layers of sludge that had accumulated in mind and body that were hampering my ability to see and be seen. I am often asked what was it that did it. What broke the cycle of illness? The truth is, there is no one thing, because Ayurveda is a whole mindbody experience. We tend to look for that simple cause and effect magic bullet, but healing is an experience of evolution and growth and — just like the growth of a plant — healing happens in many directions at once through a confluence of conditions. For myself, Ayurveda made its entrance about the same time that meditation did, and I can't tease them apart. Happily, I don't need to, as meditation is considered an integral part of Ayurveda and the two practices are beautifully inter-enhancing.

About a year before I started my personal exploration into Ayurveda, I went on my first yoga and meditation retreat and discovered meditation. Not just the moments of relaxation and calm in *shavasana* I had learned to cherish, but a real taste of another way to live in this world. I experienced a new way to relate to everything. This simple shift in perspective from being lost and caught up in unconscious thought, to noticing and observing with real-time curiosity changed my world. It felt like the first time I put on a pair of glasses at age six and suddenly everything was focused, bright, alive. There were many shades of green on that tree! I felt for the first time, a real sense of "home" within and the potential for so much more. I couldn't believe what I had been missing. So, with that amazing taste still lingering, I began to practice with the deep confidence that I was on an inevitable path. Of course, a few weeks later, day-to-day reality set in and I was back to my habits and the mental and physical suffering of perpetually being sick. However the first big insight into healing came shortly thereafter.

My mind was making me sicker.

I began to see how much the anger, frustration, sadness and victimization around being sick was creating new tension in my body. I could see how the stress of these emotions was exacerbating my condition. I shifted to an inner dialogue of, "Okay, I am sick again, sh---! This is a big bummer, but I can't change reality in this particular moment. I know everything keeps changing, and this condition too will shift and change and eventually pass as all things do, so why should I make it worse with these emotions?" I was able to allow myself to feel the real sensations of "sick," like pressure in the head, a narrowing of breath, and a heavy, earth-pulling tired. They were sensations. I found them unpleasant, but I could live through them. And, although the truth of this reality limited many of the activities I loved, ultimately it could not take away what was most important — my ability to love my young daughters. I realized I could choose to relax as much as possible through a bout of sinusitis, and this definitely made the experience less torturous. Maybe, just maybe, I thought, it might help with the healing process. This turned out to be a key ingredient in shifting the dis-ease pattern and a glimpse into the wisdom of Ayurveda.

My springboard into Ayurveda was the first home panchakarma (PK) cleanse I did, guided by an Ayurvedic practitioner. It rocked my world. Not in an earthquake kind of way, but gradually, as nature itself shapes a new environment. I didn't immediately feel better — in fact, I felt awful during the cleanse and shortly thereafter. But a shift had definitely happened. I was slightly less allergic that next fall and I noticed that herbs, I had previously taken with no effect at all, were now influencing my physiology. What I learned later was that enough of the sludge-like blockages (ama) in my system had been removed, allowing herbs to be better absorbed. This in turn created a snowball effect leading

to more openness, clarity and healing. I began integrating healthy daily habits (*dinacharya*), a balancing diet and herbs from Ayurveda into my life. It was a slow process. What I recall that first year on my venture into Ayurveda was not that the sinus infections stopped, but that the moments between episodes became longer and longer. I vividly recall that first whole week that I felt "normal." For all those challenged out there with chronic illness, you know how big this is. After almost a decade, I began to remember what wellness felt like and I had hope for the first time in many years. As I began to study Ayurveda, I was formally exposed to this key concept of self-healing I had discovered on my own: *swabha paramvad* — the body naturally moves towards health and will do so at its best, when relaxed.

After that first PK, I continued to do a cleanse on my own almost every fall and spring. Having clocked in approximately a dozen home PKs, I witnessed myself transform out of the self-identified "sick girl" into a woman who feels well most of the time. Each year that I renewed the cleanse, another layer seemed to shed itself. It has been different every time I have done this amazing cleanse. Sometimes the journey has been noticeably emotional, while in others it has been intensely physical. And some cleanses have felt very subtle with a pervading layer of calm and spontaneous awareness. I have been able to experiment along the way, fine tune the protocol, add supportive practices, and adapt to the present condition of my mindbody. While varied, these experiences have left me with more clarity, sensory sharpness and connection to my true self.

After completing the Ayurvedic practitioner program at the Mount Madonna Institute, I started inviting others to join me on the cleanse, and the group cleanse became an annual and sometimes bi-annual workshop in my community. I was able to draw from the home cleanse programs of several of my teachers, including Dr. Vasant Lad, Dr. John Doulliard and Cynthia Copple. After leading group cleanse classes since 2008, it is still evolving. And, in the midst of this perpetual evolution, we offer you this beautiful gem from Ayurveda. It has been shaped by personal and client experience, and morphed to include wonderful practices in yoga, meditation, nutrition and life-coaching. One of the biggest challenges for many folks when they begin the cleanse is figuring out what to eat. Teaming up with Adrian has been a delicious match in many ways, but especially in this area, as she had already begun compiling many wonderful cleansing recipes. Her many delightful and healthy dishes are a tremendous gift to this cleanse.

This beautiful process should be available and known to everyone. While it cannot replace a guided cleanse with a practitioner or the full supportive environment of a residential PK, our intention is to provide a comprehensive guide that is effective, accessible and self-empowering. The cleanse outlined here comes from this ancient practice of panchakarma. It is deep healing. It is not a fad, a diet or quick fix. It is a profound process that can offer you a real window into well-being, a moment of clarity in body and mind that can lead to real insights, wisdom and transformation. Your mindbody is your greatest teacher. You can view this journey you are about to undertake as a pilgrimage into knowing yourself more deeply. And, through Ayurveda, we remember our own innate ability to heal.

We will be your guides on this journey — provide you with a map, and help you pack what you need for the trip. Ultimately, however, this journey is yours. We encourage you to listen to your body, your intuition, your truth. It may be that you feel the need to linger a little longer in a particular place, or maybe you need to sit something out. It is always okay to do this. Let yourself be your own best healer.

May the journey bring you ever deeper into living your truth, helping you to feel your best and clearing the body and mind enough so you are able to see the next road. May it bring you real health, which according to Ayurveda is "abiding in the self" — a real peace in living as your unique self through this body.

It's all love.

Adrian's Story

For the first 25 years of my life, I was physically and mentally very healthy. Even though I ate the Standard American Diet ("SAD") growing up, I had great energy, good mental clarity and was able to juggle many things at once. I did amazing in school, graduating fourth in my high school class of more than 300 students. I put myself through college solely on scholarships and grants, while holding down part-time jobs to pay my bills. I finally had my own kitchen, and began to explore healthy eating. After college, I moved to the other side of the country; worked two jobs; managed volunteer fund raisers; took a few yoga classes each week; and spent every weekend hiking, backpacking and rock climbing. I was in incredible mental and physical shape, and I felt on top of the world. The only adverse symptoms I experienced at that time were the emotional roller coaster that I had come to accept as normal, and the chronic yeast infections I had been having since I was 16.

Things began to change for me when I got pregnant with my daughter, who is now seven years old. Even though my health education increased as I learned about my body's changes during pregnancy, and I worked to further refine what a healthy diet entails, I wasn't feeling myself. I felt incapable, unsure and scared of life. I thought, "Me? Scared? This rock-climbing, back-packing, hanging-with-the-guys kind of girl?" It was very out of character for me, but I assumed I was adjusting to the paradigm shift that happens in becoming a parent for the first time. I thought I'd get over it.

After childbirth, my symptoms only seemed to get worse. I cried a lot ("Okay, maybe this is normal…," I thought) and it seemed like the only emotions I felt were anger, irritability and fear of not doing things right. My husband and I went through an anti-inflammatory elimination diet and I discovered I had an issue with sugar. In the beginning, I recognized my symptoms as an overgrowth of *Candida albicans*, or a yeast overgrowth. I spent two years going through "die-off" symptoms in which I didn't feel better, and usually felt worse. I jumped into a strict anti-Candida plan so quickly, I felt like I was even more out of control, confused as to what to do or eat, and frustrated that I felt like I couldn't go to potlucks and enjoy myself because I was so militaristic about my eating habits. I dreaded running into people I knew because I didn't want to talk or socialize. I couldn't think straight, and my brain was foggy. I was highly irritable, flying off the handle at very small things. My periods still didn't come back, even months after I had stopped breastfeeding my daughter. And I would overeat — even after my stomach was full, something in my brain kept asking for more until I was so full I felt sick.

Finally, I consulted with Ronly, who helped me find a more middle-way approach to diet and lifestyle. She helped me get clear on just how stressful my life was, and gave me the space to talk about what was going on for me. I began to get much better results, and felt more relaxed, confident and not so scared. Ronly's approach to Ayurveda so beautifully embraces the Vedic concept of *Sarva karmeshu madhyamam* - "In all things, follow the middle path." This was quite a shift for me, after following such a strict diet for so long. During my second seasonal cleanse with Ronly, I went deeper into my problems and discovered that my issue with sugar was more than just Candida. Many of my symptoms were the result of blood sugar imbalances, as well. This was a pivotal discovery, as balancing my blood sugar levels helped return my mental state back to center, and helped me see how crazy I had been feeling!

The Ayurvedic path to life and living has taught me so much about not only what to eat to maintain balance, but how to eat. Ayurveda also has taught me that well-being isn't a simple matter of being sick or not, but that the unwinding of disease is a process, a journey in and of itself, that requires softening, self-forgiveness and lots and lots of love. I began to understand the difference between my symptoms and their root causes, as well as a whole-person approach to feeling well.

Once I got past the major obstacles I was facing, my mind and body were ready to take on discovering a deeper level of balance. At the time of this writing, I have now been cleansing and practicing Ayurvedic habits for more than five years, continuously going deeper in my Ayurvedic education. With each cleanse, I sense that another layer of build-up is removed: my mind is more clear, my digestion is stronger and my energy is steady. My emotional state

is more balanced than it has ever been. As my physical health continues to improve, I am also more capable of functioning in loving, deep relationships with my husband, our daughter, my sisters, my parents and my friends. Through deep personal exploration and rituals I am slowly, organically birthing layers of myself, pulling each one up, examining it and welcoming it into my consciousness.

Years ago I would have argued that it was the food alone that made such significant changes in my mindbody. However, through my formal studies in Ayurvedic medicine, my keen awareness of my experiences and my mentorship with Ronly, I understand that innumerable subtleties in life impact my mental, emotional, spiritual and physical well-being. Ayurveda teaches us that we consume everything that we come into contact with — every sight, sound, taste, touch and smell — from movies and music to food and physical contact with an animal, another human or even an inanimate object. Ayurveda has taught me to be conscious and aware of my surroundings and my mindbody and, through this awareness, to understand what I need in order to maintain balance, even on a minute scale.

My wish for this book is that it will help you gain some insight into the powerfully deep teachings of Ayurveda that I myself am just getting to know. My goal is to share as skillfully as possible about what I have learned, so that you are empowered with the tools you need for a positive journey toward balance.

Namasté.

PART I
PRINCIPLES OF AYURVEDA AND PANCHAKARMA

Chapter 1
The Ground of Ayurveda

"Ayurveda is a science of unfolding truth and as a path of discovery it has not and will not remain static."

– Sebastian Pole, Ayurvedic Medicine

UNIQUE QUALITIES OF PANCHAKARMA

Cleansing has become "a thing." Everybody is doing it. We are beginning to truly recognize our need to clear the body of toxins, and we have now accepted the ancient Ayurvedic principle that what we eat, we become. When embarking on a cleansing journey, it is important to know what your chosen method is offering you and your body. The home cleanse outlined in this book is based on traditional *panchakarma* methods from ancient Ayurveda. The process is over 2,000 years old and offers numerous benefits to the mindbody that are not addressed in many other modern cleansing methods. You will learn more about traditional panchakarma later on in this chapter. The following are some of the unique qualities offered by the ancient panchakarma (PK) method you will be using in your cleanse.

A Complete Mindbody Approach

The PK method offers more than cleansing to the physical body. It effectively removes mental, emotional and energetic imbalances as well. What this means is that there is more to this cleanse than just what you eat. We have identified three specific branches of the panchakarma process that you will be integrating into your routine during this cleanse. *Each of these are equally important.* Throughout the book, you will be guided in the most appropriate therapies from each branch to make the most out of your cleanse. The three branches are:

- Diet and Herbs
- Stress Management
- Self-Care

You can read more about these three branches in Chapter 3.

Removing Fat-Soluble Toxins with *Ghee*

Many popular cleanses in our culture are focused on clearing the digestive tract. While it is useful and beneficial to rest the digestive system, this approach does not pull the fat-soluble toxins out of the deeper tissues. This is a unique quality of an Ayurvedic cleanse, and is facilitated by the use of *ghee* in the protocol, which will loosen toxins and literally transport them out of the cells.

> **Ghee** is clarified butter, in which the difficult-to-digest proteins found in milk have been filtered out. Ghee has the unique ability to penetrate into the lipid bi-layer of cells. It is also highly nutritious and beneficial for digestion, skin and organ membranes, and is anti-inflammatory. See page 108 for more on the magic of ghee.

Emotional Clearing

An amazing attribute of this cleanse is its ability to dislodge stored emotions in the body. In our culture, we are finally recognizing the intertwined nature of body and mind. However, thousands of years ago Ayurvedic *rishis* (masters of this ancient science) had the understanding that undigested emotions were stored in the deep tissues of the body.

Dr. Vasant Lad describes these emotions as becoming crystallized in the body. When one undergoes PK, the crystals of emotion begin to dissolve. Our own experiences, and observations of others undergoing the PK cleanse, has confirmed this. There is a palpable sense of released emotions coming to the surface during the cleanse. In the process, we have the opportunity to experience feelings without getting caught up in them. We see them, observe their nuanced pattern in our bodies and actions, and we can experience them with compassion and understanding.

A More Easeful Life

This cleanse encourages and nurtures activities which are conducive to a more easeful life. We live in a very engaged, hyper-doing, success-oriented culture. This creates a lot of stress. When the mind sees the individual as separate and able to control his/her environment, there will be stress. To experience ourselves as part of a natural flow of energy in the universe, we need to have tools. In this cleanse, we will provide you with yoga and breath work for cleansing, and some simple meditation practices. These tools connect us to our source and disentangle us from the worries that lead to anxiety. Along with stress management, we will offer ideas for self-care that will support a more peaceful lifestyle. See Chapter 5 for details on these stress management practices, and Chapter 6 for self-care details.

Strengthening Digestion

Another unique feature is that we will finish the cleanse by building and strengthening our digestive capacity. By the end of the Purification Phase of the cleanse, digestion may initially become weaker, due to the increased ghee consumption and purgation. However, the Rebuilding Phase is all about increasing digestive strength. We will be applying specific Ayurvedic protocol in the immediate days following the cleanse for this purpose. During this time, we will keep to a simple diet, so that we do not overtax our digestive capacity.

You Get to Eat Real Food!

This is not a fast or a juice cleanse. The *kitchari*, or split-mung soup, that you eat as your main food during the cleanse is a complete protein. The plus, aside from the satisfaction of using your molars, is that you will have enough energy to function through a normal day. This is a very important element of a home cleanse. Traditionally, PK would be done at a retreat center away from work, kids and social activity. If you are reading this book, you are likely unable to escape from everything for two weeks to do a cleanse, and our dietary guidelines accommodate this.

Building Our Inherent Ability to Detox

Along with building digestive strength, you will also be cleaning your natural detoxification pathways, specifically the lymphatic tissue, liver and gallbladder. By doing so, you will be able to process and eliminate toxins better in the future, mitigating the build-up of toxins down the line. When our detoxification pathways are working properly, the body has the ability to detoxify on a daily basis.

Removing Toxic Build-up

Both the intestinal tract and the liver get overloaded by toxins, such as undigested food, negative emotions and environmental toxins. By eating plenty of fiber, especially from vegetables, during the Preparation and Rebuilding Phases, you are offering your intestinal tract roughage that begins to scrub the intestinal walls. By limiting fat intake, you are giving your liver a much needed rest, as the liver's job is to produce bile and digest fats. The Preparation and Rebuilding foods such as raw, grated beets, all-vegetable soups and vegetable juices, are power foods for removing toxins. They also remove excess mucus from the intestinal tract. Raw beets are especially beneficial for the liver, as they promote bile production. During the Purification Phase, the diet rich in ghee and kitchari will continue to pull toxins from the intestinal wall. You can also add bitter roots, like turmeric, dandelion and Oregon grape, which are excellent foods to detoxify the liver. Turmeric also pulls toxins from the intestinal walls.

Soothing and Repairing the Gut Lining

After toxins are removed from the lining of the intestinal walls, it is important to soothe and repair that crucial tissue. When toxic build-up occurs, the villi, or small hair-like projections that line the intestinal tract get matted down. Healthy villi are essential to absorb vital nutrients from the food you eat, strengthen the immune system and remove toxins. Eating a mono-diet of primarily (or all) kitchari is a very powerful way to soothe and rebuild the intestinal lining, both because the digestive tract can rest and because ghee and kitchari produce butyric acid, which supports the health of the colon and intestinal wall. Turmeric, added to kitchari and taken in the form of supplements, repairs the villi and soothes inflammation in the gut.

Properly Eliminating Toxins

After build up is removed from the intestinal tract and liver, it is absolutely essential that we fully remove these toxins from the body. A laxative and/or *basti* (enema therapy) near the end of the Purification Phase ensures the toxins move out.

Replenishing the Good Gut Bacteria

Adding probiotics at the end of the cleanse; continuing to use ghee in your food; and eating sprouts, greens and other high-chlorophyll foods will repopulate the beneficial intestinal microbes. This keeps digestion going strong long after your cleanse is over, strengthens your immunity and ensures problematic microbes, like yeast, do not become over-populated.

The Experience

Aside from all of the unique qualities already outlined, you may experience may other enjoyable results from this cleanse. These are:

- Clarity of senses
- Feeling lighter
- Clearer, glowing skin
- Greater presence
- Diminishing or cessation of pain, allergies, rashes
- Decreased or elimination of menstrual difficulty

- Increased energy and vibrancy
- Greater equanimity and peace

While many of these cleansing effects are experiential (that is, they are difficult to quantify, but make a significant difference in daily life), modern research has also identified further benefits of the Ayurvedic method of cleansing. In a paper by Robert E. Herron, PhD, and John B. Fagan, PhD, an Ayurvedic detoxification program — including therapies such as oleation, purgation, herbal steam baths, herbal oil massage, herbal enemas, herbal supplements and a light diet using no oils, fats or meats — was tested for effects on the mind and body. What they found was:

- Sharp reductions in total cholesterol and lipid peroxide levels
- Reduction in 14 fat-soluble toxins, such as heavy metals and pesticides (PCBs, TNC, DDE and HCB), which have been linked to endocrine disruption, developmental disorders, reproductive dysfunction, suppressed immune function, neurological problems, liver damage, dermatological disorders and cancer
- Lowered diastolic blood pressure
- Reduced state anxiety (a measure of chronic stress)

THE HISTORY OF AYURVEDA

Ayurveda has a long and rich history and is possibly the oldest system of healing known to humankind. It is the original medical system of India, and has its roots in the oldest layer of Sanskrit literature called the Vedas, which are dated between 1700-1100 BCE. The Sanskrit word *veda* means wisdom or knowledge. These texts were said to be derived from *rishis*, or seers who had direct inspiration from spiritual practice. Specifically, the early seeds of Ayurveda can be found in the *Rigveda* and *Atharvaveda*, where both healing through ritual and herbs are found, respectively. However, the first cohesive text of Ayurveda is found in the *Charaka Samhita*, dated between 150 BCE -100 CE, and is one of the three original resources for Ayurveda, with *Sushruta Samhita* and *Ashtangahrdaya Samhita* completing the triad.

Two pervading thoughts developed out of the Vedic tradition and formed the basis of Ayurveda. The first — ritual, devotion to divinities and mantra could be used in healing; the second — plants, food, herbs, minerals and direct experience could be used to treat and heal disease. Ayurveda continued to evolve in a culture that was closely linked to nature and its rhythms through an agricultural society. It evolved through practitioners and collective experience, while absorbing aspects of the developing philosophies and practices along the way, such as Yoga, Tantra, Sankhya and Buddhism.

The two Vedic streams, spiritual and experiential, are beautifully intertwined in modern Ayurveda. Its spiritual roots are interwoven into an experiential model of science based on plants, natural rhythms and universal qualities of nature. This can be seen in the way Sankhya philosophy (the influential philosophy of yoga and Ayurveda) derives the five elements, or *pancha mahabhutas*. The five elements of space, air, fire, water and earth are used to describe everything in the universe, including the human constitution, imbalances and functioning principles. In Sankhya, the elements are a result of the evolution of consciousness into matter. In this paradigm, we are all expressions of universal consciousness flowing through a particular variation of matter described by the elements and the qualities inherent in them. One of the beautiful things this concept points to is our universal connection to all things and one another.

Core Principles of Ayurveda

There are three core principals of Ayurveda. Understanding these core principals will provide you with a deeper understanding of your body, your relationships, the nature of others as well as this cleanse.

The first core quality of Ayurveda is the understanding that we are all made out of the same stuff (the elements) and that these elements affect us. Therefore, everything from the food you eat to the music you listen to and the company you keep affects your elemental expression on a fundamental level. These elements, in turn, can be thought of as just different forms of energy with varying qualities. The way these elements aggregate together form a unique expression through each individual. This goes beyond our physical appearance and body type to include our mental and emotional tendencies as well.

Each being is a unique and beautiful expression of nature!

As we deepen our understanding of our own elemental makeup and the elemental makeup of all things, we begin to see the flowing connection of energy throughout the universe. This is a very pragmatic, yet profound and verifiable way, to feel our connection with each other and nature. In other words, we are intimately connected as human beings as a continuous flow of energy, which takes shape in a temporary vessel, be it as a human, tree or eggplant.

The path to healing is a balancing act between the elemental qualities within and those in our environment. Everything is made out of the elements and the qualities inherent in them. Each element has distinct qualities and we are affected by these qualities, which we absorb from our environment. It follows then that when we take in a specific quality through our senses, it increases that same quality in our own form. And, conversely, when we take in qualities that are opposite to the ones that are in excess, we will bring the body into equilibrium. For example, if we are feeling dry — with dry skin, dry colon (constipation), etc. — and we take in dried foods, like pretzels, chips or crackers, we will increase the dry quality and tip the scales into a greater imbalance. On the other hand, if we take in moist foods, like avocados, okra, ghee, soups and liquids, the dry quality will be lessened by the opposing quality.

Additionally, these same elements have a cyclical nature in time, thus affecting the energetic qualities of the times of day, seasons and the female menstrual cycle. Therefore, living in tune with the elemental cycles keeps us connected to nature and helps us to live with more innate energy and vitality because we are going *with* the energetic flow instead of fighting against it.

The second main characteristic of Ayurveda is *swabow paramvad*: The concept that the body is always moving towards balance and does so most effectively when it is relaxed. This is mirrored in Western science, as well. The Western concept of allostasis states that there is an innate physiological movement of the body and mind towards stability and homeostasis. It is currently recognized in both the East and the West, that this state of balance is deterred by stress and struggle, and encouraged by a relaxed state.

Third, Ayurveda goes a step further in its assumption that we are, as the true tenants of our body home, our own best doctor. This is an empowering concept. We can have a profound effect on our well-being by living in accordance with nature; we are not simply hostages of our own genetic makeup. As Western medicine is discovering through epigenetics, what we eat, how we live and how we think affect how certain genes are expressed. This is totally in accordance with Ayurveda, which demonstrates that as we fine-tune our understanding of what balances our individual makeup, we move towards our original unique configuration of elements. In this way, we can become true and full versions of ourselves.

To summarize, Ayurveda is an ever-evolving science that is completely holistic. It views the body as an expression of consciousness with universal qualities that can be balanced by, and through, our environment. Our bodies have a natural intelligence that moves toward health and we are empowered to know and act on wise paths to wellness.

THE MOTHER CLEANSE: TRADITIONAL PANCHAKARMA

The Mindbody Cleanse is inspired by the ancient and profound cleansing and rejuvenation process from Ayurveda, known as *panchakarma* (PK). In this chapter, we provide some background on the fundamentals of traditional PK to provide more depth and understanding before you begin your home cleanse.

The traditional protocol of PK involves being cared for in-residence, away from normal worldly concerns and responsibilities. This is done for at least a week, but sometimes for as long as 42 days. Daily Ayurvedic body work therapies are applied with copious amounts of herbal oils to calm and nourish the nervous system. Simple, easy-to-digest, healthy meals are prepared for the person undergoing the cleanse, and there is ample time for rest, yoga and meditation. With all these things in place, it is easy to imagine how the body and mind could finally be able to really let go. The channels of the body open and soften, and the sticky, dense nature of ama liquefies and is eliminated, leaving the channels unobstructed and clear. The patterns of thoughts and emotions are freed up and we are able to witness them as simply habitual thought patterns, without confusing ourselves with them.

The aim of PK is to clear the mind and body of these toxins, referred to as *ama* in Ayurveda. Most modern cleanses simply clear the digestive system, while PK goes beyond this by pulling deep-seated, fat-soluble toxins from the body and old, unprocessed emotions from the mind. In PK, the body is properly prepared for detoxification, creating a much more thorough cleanse with long-lasting results. Additionally, the whole mindbody is transformed to prevent further build-up of toxins through clearing of the natural detox pathways — the liver and lymph — and rebuilding digestive strength. Once obstructions are cleared from the body, energy flows more freely. As a result, the inherent intelligence of the mindbody can facilitate deep healing and allow us to live up to our potential.

The word panchakarma literally means the "five actions," and refers to the therapies used to rid the body of ama. Although the literal translation of PK refers to these five specific actions, the term *panchakarma* is used to describe a complete detoxification and rejuvenation process with three parts:

Part 1 is *purvakarma* and can be thought of as the preparation of the mindbody for the removal of toxins. (In The Mindbody Cleanse, this includes the 4-day Preparation Phase, and the first six days of the Purification Phase.)

Part 2 is *panchakarma*, the actual five therapies to remove toxins, with each therapy addressing a particular area and quality of the body. (In The Mindbody Cleanse, we do this on day(s) seven and eight of the Purification Phase.)

In Part 3, *paschatkarma* protocol is established to strengthen digestion, build immunity and nourish all the tissues of the body. (In The Mindbody Cleanse, these are the Rebuilding and Rejuvenation Phases.)

In order to fully appreciate and understand the purpose of this home cleanse, let's further explore panchakarma.

Traditional Panchakarma
PK unwinds the disease process. According to Ayurveda, disease begins in the digestive system as an imbalance. The imbalance builds, then overflows. It enters into circulation and eventually lodges in weak, vulnerable tissues of the body where it can then proliferate and mutate into various disease manifestations. This process is reversed in PK.

First, these deep-seated toxins are loosened through the oleation process during purvakarma. Oleation is the oiling and softening of the body from the inside and out. From the outside, specific types of herbal oil are massaged into the body, while from the inside, ghee is ingested in increasing amounts, becoming the chelator for fat-soluble toxins. When the cells are saturated with ghee, the fat-soluble toxins will naturally move into the higher concentration of fat particles found in the ghee. This effectively pulls out the toxins.

In conjunction with the oleation process, the body is warmed, again holistically, from the inside with digestive herbs and from the outside with steam and other heat therapies. The result: the body softens, the vessels dilate, channels throughout the cells begin to open, and the ama loosens. The loosened ama and ghee then moves back into circulation where it can be worked on by the liver, and eventually sent back to the digestive system by way of bile. Once the ama is in the digestive system, it can be more readily evacuated through PK therapies.

At this point, the therapies of PK are employed to eliminate the ama from the body. Traditionally, these five therapies include:

> - **Nasya:** herbal oil administered into the nose
> - **Vamana:** therapeutic emesis (vomiting)
> - **Virechena:** therapeutic purgation using a strong laxative
> - **Basti:** herbal enemas
> - **Raktamokshana:** therapeutic withdrawal of blood

Depending on the constitution and current state of the individual, some or all of these therapies are utilized. In the moderated home cleanse, you will only be using the therapies of purgation and enema in addition to the cleansing diet, yoga and meditation.

Paschatkarma, the Rebuilding and Rejuvenation Phases, use diet, herbs and yoga to rebuild and strengthen digestion. Once the digestive strength is back, *rasayana* herbs and foods are taken in to nourish the function and quality of all tissues of the body. *Rasayana*, or rejuvenation, comes from the words *rasa* (the juice or essence of life), and *ayana* (the path). Therefore, rasayana is the path to rejuvenation and longevity. It is that which nourishes all seven tissue systems of the body. It follows the panchakarma cleanse, as the food and herbs taken in the Rejuvenation Phase are nourishing and building in nature. It is important to do rasayana therapies *following* panchakarma because the body must be prepared to fully receive and absorb these herbs and foods. Digestion must be strong enough, blockages in the body removed, and the body's functioning principles balanced. This is truly the most beneficial part of the Ayurvedic cleanse. In fact, Ayurveda views the cleanse process as simply a preparation for rejuvenation.

The elegance of panchakarma lies in its complete process. By preparing the body through oleation, eliminating the toxins from the gastro-intestinal tract and finally, rebuilding the tissues through rejuvenation, the mindbody is deeply cleansed and the doshas, energetic principles, are brought into balance.

Chapter 2
Understanding Your Unique Constitution

There is vitality,
a life force that is translated through you into action.
And because there is only one of you in all time,
this expression is unique, and if you block it,
it will never exist through any other medium and be lost.
It is not your business to determine how good it is,
or how valuable it is,
or how it compares with others' expressions.
It is your business to keep it yours,
to keep the channel open.
You do not even have to believe
in yourself or your works.
You have to keep an open mind
and be aware directly to the urges that motivate you.

- Martha Graham

As you learned in Chapter 1, Ayurveda is truly a holistic system. Ayurveda teaches us that everything is made of the five elements: air, space, fire, water and earth. These elements are found in nature, in our food, in our bodies — in everything. Rather than treating symptoms, it aims to treat the whole person, and understanding your unique constitution, or mindbody type, is essential in this process.

Your *Prakruti*
The elements you were born with
Your individual constitution is referred to as your *prakruti* in Ayurveda, and this indicates the unique combination of elements at the time you were born. Your prakruti is based on your parents' prakrutis and the elements that were present in the surrounding environment at the moment you were conceived. For example, if your parents are both dominantly *kapha* (earth and water) and you are conceived during spring (a season dominated by kapha), you are likely to be very kapha-dominant. If both of your parents have *pitta* (fire and water) in their constitution and you are conceived in a passionate or fiery situation, or during summer (a season dominated by pitta), you will be born with a significant amount of pitta in your constitution.

It is important not to stereotype yourself into a constitutional type. The way the elements present themselves in each person is completely unique. Two people can both be pitta-dominant, with *vata* (space and air) as a secondary presenting element, but one may be physically very hot and have the mental "spaciness" of vata, while the other may have the short temper of pitta, and the cold hands and feet of vata. Pay attention to how the elements present themselves in you, and begin to notice how they play out in others. In this way, you can begin to better understand yourself and the people around you.

Your *Vikruti*
Your elements in the current moment
While your prakruti does not change throughout life, you can become imbalanced. Emotional, spiritual and environmental factors may affect the expression of the qualities in you. Because of this, Ayurveda also recognizes an individual's *vikruti*, which is the expression of elements in your mind and body in the current moment. This is where imbalance shows up. This snapshot can give valuable insight into what you can do right now to bring yourself back into balance.

Your vikruti is ever-changing. It is like an energetic river, always flowing and moving. Bringing your awareness to your vikruti, or how you are in each moment, is a beautiful way you can utilize Ayurvedic wisdom in your daily life. Seeing and understanding when a quality is out of balance gives you insight into how to get back to the true, harmonious nature you were born with. When an element is out of balance, you will notice because you are no longer functioning optimally. The word *dosha* means "fault." If you can become aware of and acknowledge faults and imbalances, you can work with Ayurvedic principles — using food and lifestyle habits — to bring yourself back into balance. This re-calibration of elements can be very powerful in the initial stages of imbalance by preventing disease from taking root.

The Importance of Balancing Vata

For most people, the vata dosha will tend to go out of balance the most. In general, the environment of our culture is highly vata-aggravating. This is because our value system tends to promote doing and accomplishing as much as possible, even if it means pushing the mind and body into over exertion. Additionally, we are constantly bombarded by information and exposed to sensory stimulation. All of this puts a strain on our nervous system, which is considered predominately a vata function because of its subtle movement throughout the body. It is important to keep vata balanced because the nervous system governs all of the other systems and doshas.

Assessing Your Constitution

While some people can identify a single dosha as dominant in their constitution, some people show two doshas more or less equal. For example, a person who shows pitta as their strongest dosha with vata being a close second, would be considered a pitta-vata constitution. This is different than a vata-pitta constitution, where a person is primarily of a vata type, with pitta showing up secondarily. Although rare, in some cases all three doshas are fairly equal within one person.

In the charts on the following pages, make a check mark next to each of the qualities that describe you at this time. (Remember, your constitution in this moment is likely different than that as a child, or even that of last year.) Add up the number of qualities from each category to determine which elements are most prominent for you right now. Keep the numbers of your "In Balance" answers separate from your "Out of Balance" answers so you can see which element is most out of balance. You may want to pay special attention to the out-of-balance element during your cleanse.

You can try this exercise several times, using a different color check mark for each time period:

- The course of your life — an "overall picture" (this will be most similar to your prakriti)
- The past year
- The past month
- Today

When answering based on the recent past, pay attention to the imbalances you notice to get an idea of your vikruti, and what imbalances need to be addressed currently.

(Keep in mind: only so much can be gained from a quiz. This is not meant to be a thorough assessment. It is useful to see an Ayurvedic practitioner for a more complete and accurate sense of your personal makeup.)

Vata - Air and Space

Because vata is dominated by air and space, people with a strong vata constitution may be referred to as "spacey" or indecisive. The word "changeable" is a good description of the vata-type person, as they have irregular patterns in sleeping, eating and digestion. Vatas tend to be creative. They also walk and talk fast. Physically, they tend to have a thin, bony frame. Much of the work of balancing vata is slowing down, connecting to the earth and resting often. Heavy, oily, moist and dense foods like avocados, nuts and seeds, and cooked vegetables are best for vatas. Light and dry foods, such as crackers, rice cakes and dry cereals may bring vata even further out of balance.

In Balance	Out of Balance

Mental Tendencies

In Balance	Out of Balance
☐ Excited	☐ Light sleeper
☐ Creative, artistic	☐ Tires easily
☐ Imaginative	☐ Erratic speech
☐ Alert, clear-minded	☐ Fast talking
☐ Spontaneous	☐ Thinking too much
☐ Mentally flexible	☐ "Spacey"
☐ Grasps new ideas quickly	☐ Disorganized
☐ Quick	☐ Poor memory
☐ Enjoys plays, stories, jokes; funny	☐ Indecisive
	☐ Quickly changing thoughts

Emotional Tendencies

In Balance	Out of Balance
☐ Adaptable	☐ Fear, anxiety, worry
☐ Very perceptive	☐ Depression
☐ Compassionate	☐ Easily hurt
☐ Aware of subtle energies	☐ Judgmental
☐ Joyful, happy	☐ Moody
	☐ Impatient

Spiritual Tendencies

In Balance	Out of Balance
☐ Very spiritual	☐ Variable faith
☐ Intuitive, clairvoyant	☐ Feels ungrounded
☐ Many dreams	

	In Balance	**Out of Balance**

Physical Tendencies

In Balance	Out of Balance
☐ Thin frame	☐ Underweight
☐ Tall or short	☐ Dry hair/nails/skin
☐ Small eyes, often dark	☐ Dry constipation
☐ Thin, small nose	☐ Variable appetite
☐ Coarse or thin hair	☐ Weak stomach
☐ Long neck	☐ Restless, can't sit still
☐ Prominent veins	☐ Cold hands/feet
☐ Small teeth and gums	☐ Insomnia
☐ Enjoys vigorous exercise	☐ Easily fatigued
☐ Walks quickly	☐ Low back ache
☐ Irregular hunger and digestion	☐ Gas, bloating
☐ Prefers warm, humid weather	

Relationship Tendencies

In Balance	Out of Balance
☐ Outgoing, social	☐ Shy and introverted
☐ Many casual relationships	☐ Poor self-esteem
☐ Strong communicator	☐ Interrupts
☐ Charismatic	☐ Zones out in conversation
	☐ Insecure
	☐ Fear of commitment

	In Balance	**Out of Balance**
Vata Totals		

Pitta - Fire and Water

The pitta-type person is often described as intense. Pitta's fire shows up as drive, passion and motivation, but can quickly turn into over-working or perfectionism. They are natural leaders and can be very organized. However, when out of balance, pittas can become controlling or overly competitive. Physically, pitta-types are hot, with a medium build and often very athletic. The work of balancing pitta involves cooling down and taking time to play more. Cooling foods balance pitta, such as cilantro and cucumber, while spicy-hot foods may exacerbate pitta.

In Balance	Out of Balance

Mental Tendencies

☐ Ambitious	☐ Loud
☐ Organized, great planner	☐ Egotistical
☐ Sharp memory	☐ Workaholic
☐ Logical	☐ Creates problems that don't exist
☐ Problem solver	☐ Overactive mind
☐ Very orderly	☐ Perfectionist
☐ Inventive	☐ Controlling
☐ Goal-oriented	
☐ Decisive	
☐ Strong willpower, when decides to	

Emotional Tendencies

☐ Joyful	☐ Angry, irritable
☐ Observant of others' emotions	☐ Demeaning
☐ Adventurous	☐ Competitive to a fault
☐ Passionate	☐ Suppresses emotions
	☐ Fear of failure
	☐ Reckless

Spiritual Tendencies

☐ Intensely spiritual	☐ Extremist
☐ Determined	☐ Materialistic
☐ Leader	☐ Cynical
☐ Appreciates beauty	☐ Desires power

	In Balance	Out of Balance

Physical Tendencies

In Balance	Out of Balance
☐ Medium build	☐ Acne
☐ Medium height	☐ Skin rashes
☐ Thin, pointed nose	☐ Diarrhea
☐ Eyes medium-sized, penetrating	☐ Profuse perspiration
☐ Strong appetite	☐ Strong body odor
☐ Walks with determination	☐ Inflammation
☐ Sharp, direct speech	☐ Indigestion, ulcers
☐ Freckles, moles	☐ Heartburn, acid reflux
☐ Reddish or brown hair	☐ Easily overheated
☐ Sound sleeper	
☐ High body temperature	
☐ Prefers cool weather, adverse to very hot weather	

Relationship Tendencies

In Balance	Out of Balance
☐ Charismatic	☐ Controlling
☐ Natural leader	☐ Overly extroverted
☐ Confident	☐ Aggressive
☐ Mostly work/business relationships	☐ Manipulative
☐ Helpful	☐ Stubborn
☐ Kind	☐ Jealous
	☐ Critical/judgmental
	☐ Compares self and others

	In Balance	Out of Balance
Pitta Totals		

Kapha - Earth and Water

Kapha's earth and water translates into a slow and steady pace, reliability, dependability and a calm demeanor. Kaphas are truly "like the water" — they let things roll off their backs and "go with the flow." They have the most stamina and strongest memory of all of the mindbody types. Physically, they tend to have a heavier frame with big bones and tend toward weight gain (although all body types can become overweight when imbalanced). When out of balance, kaphas may become lethargic, depressed or possessive. The work of balancing kapha involves getting plenty of physical activity and varying the routine. Kaphas do best with foods that are light, such as plenty of vegetables and lower fat foods, while avoiding those that are heavy or mucus-producing, such as heavy animal protein, wheat, dairy and sugars.

In Balance	Out of Balance
Mental Tendencies	
☐ Calm, steady	☐ Lethargic
☐ Excellent memory	☐ Over-sleeping
☐ Very present	☐ Overly passive
☐ Clear thinking	☐ Slow to understand things
☐ Completes projects	☐ Stuck in routine
☐ Methodical	☐ Attached to material possessions
Emotional Tendencies	
☐ Very stable	☐ Unable to express oneself
☐ Slow to change	☐ Depression
☐ Considerate	☐ Addictions
☐ Sentimental	☐ "Stuck in a rut"
☐ Good-natured	☐ Overly sensitive
Spiritual Tendencies	
☐ Satisfied with life	☐ Greedy
☐ Deep, abiding faith	☐ Possessive
☐ Conservative	☐ Fear of letting go
	☐ Complacent

	In Balance	Out of Balance

Physical Tendencies

In Balance	Out of Balance
☐ Broad frame	☐ Obese or overweight
☐ Strong	☐ Gives up easily
☐ Well proportioned	☐ Slow digestion
☐ Thick hair, often dark, wavy or curly	☐ Slow metabolism
☐ Smooth, lustrous skin	☐ Oily skin
☐ Large, thick nose	☐ Water retention
☐ Large doe-like eyes	☐ Congestion, mucus
☐ Melodious voice	☐ Sinus infection
☐ Moderate appetite	☐ Aversion toward exercise
☐ Great stamina	☐ Laziness
☐ Deep sleeper	
☐ Graceful	
☐ Prefers warm, dry climate	

Relationship Tendencies

In Balance	Out of Balance
☐ Patient, loving	☐ Jealous
☐ Forgiving	☐ Unable to say no
☐ Slow speech, few words	☐ Easily taken advantage of
☐ Desire to help others	☐ Takes on others' problems
☐ Loyal, attached	☐ Introverted
☐ Nurturing	☐ Difficulty letting go
☐ Accepting	
☐ Romantic	
☐ Community oriented	
☐ Long, deep relationships	
☐ Good listener	

	In Balance	Out of Balance
Kapha Totals		

Mindbody Type Totals

	In Balance	Out of Balance	Total
Vata			
Pitta			
Kapha			

So What Does This Mean For Me?

After adding up totals for each dosha, take a look at where the highest numbers are. If you have a high number in both columns of a particular dosha, it is safe to assume you have a lot of that dosha in your constitution. If you have an area where there is a significant number of tendencies in the "Out of Balance" category, you can adjust your cleanse protocol (see page 101-102) and work on bringing this into balance after the cleanse.

Remember: This is a basic snapshot of how you are right now. You are always changing, like a flowing river – seasonally, daily or even by the minute. To label yourself pitta and decide you will never eat spicy food again is missing the point. Ayurvedic theory can empower you to find balance in each moment, and therefore to have a greater picture of your life. The empowering piece of this is noticing and understanding the current imbalanced doshas. This offers, in real time, an amazing, natural tool to help you re-align your health.

By tuning in daily to the messages your body is giving you throughout the cleanse, you can become practiced at noticing which elements are out of balance. This will be a great spring-board into self-empowered healing through Ayurveda.

Balance Using The Elements

Understanding the elements, their qualities and how they manifest in a living being can be a valuable map to staying healthy. The tendencies found in each constitutional type are a reflection of how these elements manifest. For example, the air and space of vata can manifest as being spacey and unfocused, while the fire element of pitta can manifest as being passionate. As you become acquainted with these elements, you will begin to notice their presence in your mindbody at different times, and how they correlate to the tendencies of your dosha. Getting back in the driver's seat on your journey to health means regularly checking in with yourself to find out what elements are at play - which ones are in balance and which ones need some help re-balancing. While a practitioner or book can support you in discovering ways of coming back into balance, no one knows your body like you do. You are the key to your own well-being.

Paying attention to the environment around you is also important in maintaining balance. Ayurveda teaches us that each season carries a preponderance of certain elements: fall and early winter are associated with vata because of cold, blowing winds; summer is associated with pitta because of the sun's heat; and kapha dominates late winter/spring because of rain and melting snow. However, even these are generalizations that are not to be taken without personal consideration! In a high-desert area, where spring brings little rain but plenty of strong, cool winds, vata will be a main influencing principle.

Like Increases Like, Opposites Balance

Ayurveda's five-element theory teaches that everything is made up of the elements and that each element is made up of several qualities. These qualities (*gunas*) each have a corresponding opposite quality. A principle teaching of Ayurveda is that you can re-balance the mindbody by taking in the opposite quality of the imbalanced one. It is very pragmatic. When you are noticing a quality, it is a sign that it has become overly abundant. For example, if you notice dry bowels (constipation), you can assume that there is too much dry quality. By taking in the opposite — the moist/wet quality — you bring the body back to equilibrium. This is most simply done with foods and beverages, but can also be done with herbs and lifestyle practices.

We encourage you to focus on the *qualities* in you, your environment and your food. Understanding this is far more useful than pegging yourself as a certain mindbody type and eating one doshic diet all year long. The practice of finding balance is dynamic. By staying present and noticing your environment and the subtle qualities present in your mindbody, you will be able to make adjustments day-to-day. This will facilitate finding balance more quickly, before imbalanced doshas can take root as dis-ease. This illustrates the need to be keenly aware of how you are feeling, as our bodies are always changing in response to our food, environment and surroundings.

The charts on the following pages list different qualities you may find in yourself, your food or your surroundings. Note that these qualities are not "bad" — it is when they are in excess that they become a problem. To the right of each quality you find suggested foods or activities you can use to bring yourself back into balance by applying the principle of opposites.

Balance Using the Qualities

Cold

May manifest as:

- Cold hands and feet
- Feeling cold in general
- Nervousness
- Anxiety
- Cough
- Congestion, asthma, sinus problems
- Tightness
- Muscle spasm
- Poor circulation

Ways to Balance

- Eat warm, cooked foods
- Take saunas and baths often
- Surround yourself with warm colors, such as reds, oranges and yellows
- Massage yourself with warm oil daily
- Sunbathe
- Drink plenty of warm or hot filtered water
- Choose warming spices, such as cinnamon, cloves, fresh ginger, garlic and black pepper

Dry

May manifest as:

- Dry skin, hair, lips or nails
- Constipation, dry or hard stools
- Bloating, gas
- Dehydration

Ways to Balance

- Eat oily, moist, cooked foods, such as soups and stews with good oil
- Drink plenty of warm or hot filtered water
- Practice self-abhyanga daily using a good quality oil, such as sesame

Light

May manifest as:

- Feeling "spacey"
- Dizziness, feeling light-headed
- Nervousness, anxiety, restlessness
- Talking or walking extremely fast
- Thinness, weight-loss
- Insomnia
- Sensitivity to light and heat
- Ringing in ears

Ways to Balance

- Eat dense, oily foods, such as avocados, nuts and seeds
- Include plenty of grounding root vegetables and good protein in your diet
- Spend quiet time away from activity
- Perform self-massage daily with warm oil
- Practice grounding meditations and yoga

Balance Using the Qualities

Subtle

May manifest as:

- Sensitivity
- Easily over-stimulated or excited
- Tremors, twitching
- Fear, anxiety, insecurity

Ways to Balance

- Practice grounding yoga, qigong or meditation
- Spend time gardening
- Follow a regular eating schedule

Mobile

May manifest as:

- Talking too much
- Multi-tasking without focus
- Feeling "scattered"
- Racing mind, restlessness
- Fidgeting
- Muscle twitching or palpitations
- ADD/ADHD
- Inability to complete projects

Ways to Balance

- Ground yourself with heavy foods that have plenty of good fat and oil
- Eat more root vegetables, such as carrots, beets and rutabaga
- Take on fewer commitments
- Be still — practice seated and lying meditation
- Choose gentle exercise, such as walking or slow yoga
- Travel less

Hot

May manifest as:

- Irritability, anger, impatience
- Physically feeling overheated
- Rashes or arthritis
- Heartburn or acid reflux
- Perfectionism
- Overly judgmental
- Over-working
- Excessive perspiration
- Fevers or infections
- Burning sensations (anywhere)
- Insomnia due to over-thinking

Ways to Balance

- Choose cooling foods, such as cucumber and cilantro
- Spend time in the shade or indoors during the heat of the day
- Exercise during the coolest part of the day
- Keep stress levels low
- Choose cooling colors for clothing and surroundings, such as blue, violet, green and white
- Practice surrender
- Meditate daily, or as often as possible
- Swim in cool water

Balance Using the Qualities

Oily/Wet

May manifest as:

- Oily skin or hair, acne
- Clammy skin
- Diarrhea or thick/sticky bowels
- Water retention, swelling
- Swollen joints
- Heavy mind, slow thinking

Ways to Balance

- Favor foods that are drying (astringent): lentils, beans, dried corn and quinoa
- Eat less oil and fat
- Spend time in dry places, such as dry saunas, or indoors if you live in a rainy climate

Sharp

May manifest as:

- Overly judgmental, uncompromising
- Manipulating
- Lack of compassion
- Anger or irritability
- Over-working
- Ulcers, gastritis, acid reflux
- Sharp headaches, sharp pain anywhere

Ways to Balance

- Practice loving-kindness toward self and others
- Practice relaxation and surrender
- Choose cooling foods, such as cucumber, cilantro, lime, coconut and salad
- Meditate daily, or as often as possible

Slow/Static

May manifest as:

- Oversleeping, lethargy
- Depression
- Slow digestion
- Overly passive

Ways to Balance

- Get plenty of physical activity
- Vary your routine
- Include plenty of fresh, non-starchy vegetables in your diet
- Rise before the sun in the morning
- Choose bold, energizing colors for clothing and surroundings, such as red, yellow, gold and orange

Balance Using the Qualities

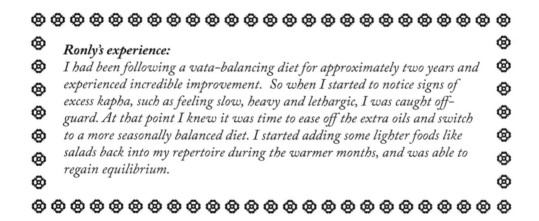

May manifest as:

- Fatigue or lethargy
- Stubbornness
- Attachment
- Weight-gain, water retention
- Congestion or sinus infection
- Stuck in a routine
- Depression
- Weak digestion, food allergies

Heavy

Ways to Balance

- Choose light foods, such as non-starchy vegetables and puffed grains
- Include some physical activity each day
- Vary your routine
- Surround yourself with colors that promote lightness in the body, such as purple and pale yellow

✿✿✿✿✿✿✿✿✿✿✿✿✿✿✿✿✿✿✿✿✿✿✿✿✿

Ronly's experience:
I had been following a vata-balancing diet for approximately two years and experienced incredible improvement. So when I started to notice signs of excess kapha, such as feeling slow, heavy and lethargic, I was caught off-guard. At that point I knew it was time to ease off the extra oils and switch to a more seasonally balanced diet. I started adding some lighter foods like salads back into my repertoire during the warmer months, and was able to regain equilibrium.

✿✿✿✿✿✿✿✿✿✿✿✿✿✿✿✿✿✿✿✿✿✿✿✿✿

PART 2
THE MINDBODY CLEANSE ESSENTIALS

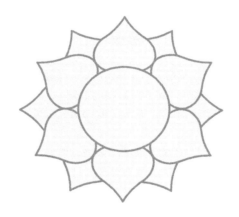

Chapter 3
Overview of the Mindbody Cleanse

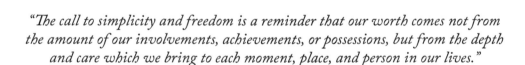

"The call to simplicity and freedom is a reminder that our worth comes not from the amount of our involvements, achievements, or possessions, but from the depth and care which we bring to each moment, place, and person in our lives."

– Richard A. Bower

You are about to begin an amazing journey. While much of what will unfold will be unique to you, we will provide you with a solid map to guide you along the way. Before getting into the detailed instructions of the cleanse in Chapter 7, lets look at the big picture—the aerial map.

The goal of the Mindbody Cleanse is to emulate as much as possible the profound process of PK, while keeping it accessible within the context of your full life. You will still be able to attend to your work and family responsibilities in our modified version. The intention is to create an environment of support and security so that you can let go and release toxic build-up and stagnant emotions.

SETTING INTENTIONS

Before you begin, it is important to set an intention for the cleanse in order to deepen the experience on many levels. For example, if your heartfelt intention is to learn to care for yourself, then by proclaiming this and formally setting that as an intention, you are already orienting your consciousness in that direction. It is like sending an invisible arrow out in that direction for your body and mind to follow. Your intention is also something you can return to if cleansing becomes difficult or uncomfortable. The simple act of taking a quiet moment to focus on your intention can help bring you back to center.

A Practice for Identifying Your Intention

Sit comfortably and feel into the body. Notice the shape of your body in space, and the feel of the hips in contact with the earth through gravity. Then, pay attention to several breaths, following closely as air moves into and out of the body; notice the feeling of the breath touching the body from the inside. Once the mind is settled on these sensations, feel into the center of the chest. Ask yourself, "What is my heartfelt intention in doing this cleanse?" Listen to what arises as you connect to your deeply held wisdom. Trust the answer or feeling sense of what comes up. In this way, you will align yourself to your deep purpose and intention.

THE THREE PHASES OF THE MINDBODY CLEANSE

The whole cleanse process will take approximately two weeks: at least four days of preparation, seven to eight days of purification, and three days for rebuilding digestion. At the end of the 14 days, you will add rejuvenating foods and herbs to your diet.

• *The Preparation Phase:* You eat a low-fat, whole foods, simple diet of foods that are easy-to-digest. We include some simple liver clearing practices and effective stress management practices, such as yoga and meditation. The Preparation Phase usually lasts four days to one week, but can be applied for up to several weeks.

• *The Purification Phase:* You eat an even simpler diet, consisting mainly of kitchari. The Purification Phase lasts seven to eight days, with PK therapies (the procedures for direct removal of ama from the digestive tract) on days seven and eight. You will be ingesting ghee in increasing amounts for 7 days. If you are vegan you can use olive oil, flax oil or a combination of these. On day seven you will take a plant-based laxative to remove the ama from the GI tract. On day eight, you have the option of continuing this through an herbal enema.

In short, the The Purification Phase includes:

- Oiling and warming the body (self-massage, baths/saunas)
- Daily ghee intake
- Eating kitchari as the main food
- Self-care (massage, journaling, acupuncture, etc.)
- Yoga, meditation and pranayama (breathing practices)
- Purgation on seventh day
- Herbal/oil enema on day eight (optional)

• *The Rebuilding and Rejuvenating Phases:* The Rebuilding Phase involves returning to the Preparation Phase diet and adding herbs and foods to build digestive strength. We will do this for at least three days. The second aspect, the Rejuvenation Phase, involves adding rejuvenating foods and herbs to nourish body tissues once digestion is strong enough for them to be incorporated into your sustainable diet.

THE THREE BRANCHES

Cleansing is about more than just food; in fact, we view diet and herbs as only one-third of the cleansing protocol. Each phase of the

Kitchari is a combination of split mung beans, rice and spices, of which we provide delicious variations and adjustments to fit your needs! It is easy to digest, nutritious and conducive to removing ama. See page 106 for more information on why kitchari is an ideal cleansing food, or see pages 231 - 237 for kitchari recipes.

Ayurvedic home cleanse will include three specific, and equally important, branches. You will incorporate aspects of each of these into all phases of cleansing. These are:

• *Diet and Herbs* - Throughout the three phases of this cleanse you will be eating a simplified, whole foods diet. During the Purification Phase, the diet is simplified further and is mainly composed of kitchari. Kitchari is a very important part of removing toxic build-up and is soothing and healing to the intestinal tract. To this simple diet, you can add herbs (optionally) to support digestion, elimination, lymphatic flow, liver health and blood-sugar regulation. Because Ayurvedic herbs are generally whole herbs, they are considered a dietary component.

• *Stress Management* - This branch is composed of yoga, pranayama (breath work) and meditation. See Chapter 5 for details on these practices. While we put more emphasis on these practices during the Purification Phase, it is most effective to incorporate them into all phases of the cleanse. These practices may prove to be so beneficial that you find yourself continuing them after the cleanse.

• *Self-Care* - This branch centers on creating a supportive lifestyle for the cleanse. The focus is on limiting activity, clearing space in your schedule, and daily self-massage (abhyanga), which can be followed by a hot bath, shower or sauna. The daily abhyanga is one of the unique aspects of an Ayurvedic cleanse, and supports the release of toxins stored in fat cells. This practice also calms the nervous system, further promoting stress management. There are many other self-care options, as outlined on page 83, and we hope you are able to use some of these to support your cleanse.

The charts on the following pages give a basic overview of what your cleansing schedule will look like.

Preparation Phase - 4 Days

Diet and Herbs:
- Eat a diet that is low-fat, whole foods and seasonal. (See Chapter 7 for specifics.)
- Drink fresh squeezed vegetable and fruit juices, especially apple juice and green vegetable juices. Fresh is best, but Odwalla and Naked brands work, too.
- Eat lots of vegetables to scrub the intestinal lining. Cooked vegetables are easiest to digest. Eat a portion of Beet Liver Cleanser (page 165) with meals.
- Take a Liver Flush Smoothie (page 145) once during Preparation Phase.
- Start your herbal regimen on day 1 of the Preparation Phase, if choosing to take any supplemental herbs.
- Balance your blood sugar levels by including fiber and protein (vegetables, whole grains, legumes) in your meals, and by eating enough at each meal to last until the next meal.
- Continue taking all medications.

Stress Management:
- Practice 10-15+ minutes of yoga, meditation, pranayama or any combination of these each morning before breakfast, or whenever you can work it into your schedule.

Self-Care:
- Take some extra time for yourself in whatever way feels most relaxing to you. Some ideas are walking in nature, hot baths, extra meditation or prayer time, or extra sleep.
- Plan to cook more than usual during the Preparation Phase. Because the diet does not include any oils with meals, it may be difficult to eat out.

Purification Phase - 7-8 Days

Diet and Herbs:
- Eat a primarily kitchari diet. (See pages 105 - 107 for meal options and pages 228 - 237 for recipes.)
- Take melted ghee each morning on an empty stomach. (See page 107 for schedule). Wait until you feel hunger before eating anything else (at least 15 minutes).
- Drink the purgative on Day 7 of the Purification Phase. If possible, take this between 10am and 2pm on an empty stomach, or at least 2 hours after eating.
- Administer an enema on Day 8 (optional).
- Continue taking all medications.
- Continue taking any herbs for the cleanse.
- Stop taking any supplements that are not part of the cleanse, if you feel you can go without them. If you normally take fish, flax or borage oil capsules and feel you cannot go without them, take them with the morning ghee.

Stress Management:
- Practice 10-15+ minutes of pranayama, yoga and/or meditation daily.

Self-Care:
- Include a self-oil massage before a hot bath, shower or sauna daily.

* Schedule Days 7 and 8 of the Purification Phase at a time when you can be at home relaxing because of the purgative and basti on these days.

Rebuilding Phase - 3 Days *(or more – until digestion feels strong again)*	
Diet and Herbs: • Follow the Digestive Reset protocol (see page 119) using lemon, ginger and herbs. • Continue following the simplified diet utilized during the Preparation Phase. • Continue taking herbs and supplements for the cleanse until they are gone. • Add probiotic foods and/or supplements to repopulate beneficial bacteria.	**Stress Management:** • Practice 10-15+ minutes of pranayama, yoga and/or meditation daily. **Self-Care:** • Spend the first day of this phase relaxing at home.

Rejuvenation Phase - 7 days to 3 months *(this will merge into your Maintenance Diet)*	
Diet and Herbs: • Add rejuvenating foods and herbs (see pages 124 - 125). • Continue to focus on strengthening digestion. • Continue taking herbs and supplements for the cleanse until they are gone	**Stress Management:** • Continue to practice 10-15 minutes of yoga, stretching, meditation and/or prayer in the morning, or whenever it fits into your day. **Self-Care:** • As you return to your maintenance diet and lifestyle, choose one or two self-care practices that you particularly enjoyed to integrate into your daily routine.

HOW TO SCHEDULE YOUR CLEANSE

Imagine your body beginning to detox: ama (toxic build-up) begins to loosen from the organs and move into the bloodstream. While this is happening, your body will be working on metabolizing as much of these toxins as possible. While doing this extra processing, the body may feel tired at times. Additionally, old, difficult emotions may begin to surface as molecules of long-held emotion become dislodged from the deeper tissues.

Now imagine this is all happening while you are running around with the usual busy schedule of work, parenting, social activities and all the other things you normally do. When we are busy, it is more difficult for the minbody to relax enough to allow for the process of letting go.

Therefore, it is important to pick a week for the purification phase that has as little demands as possible, emulating the conditions of an in-residence PK. When we create space in our schedules, we support our bodies in doing this deep work of self-healing. We will be able to better relax into the cleanse, invest in learning healthy habits and, most importantly, have time to notice what is happening. This is a huge gift. We begin to cultivate awareness of how our habits, food and emotional patterns affect us. In this awareness, wisdom has an opportunity to grow and help us evolve. The journey may present us with challenges and, if we have more easeful conditions, we will find we are more clear, sane and less crabby as we work through them.

For women, you should make an effort to schedule your home cleanse so as not to coincide with menstruation. Of course, sometimes this will happen anyway, and you can make adjustments to your protocol. See pages 116 - 117 for tips on how to adjust your cleanse during menstruation.

Finally, you will want to make sure that the day you take your purgative (day 7 of the Purification Phase) is free so you can be at home relaxing. If you choose to do the enema on day 8, you will want to have extra time at home to prepare and administer it at a relaxed pace.

Tips for Clearing Space

You will be spending more time than usual on self-care, sleep, meals and quiet contemplation or meditation during your cleanse. Give yourself permission to do so. Once the cleanse is over you can return to your usual schedule but we hope you will welcome one or two of your favorite techniques into your daily or weekly rituals.

Through this process, take note of any underlying thoughts or emotions that arise during your self-care and quiet time. Some common themes that may arise are:

- "I should be doing…"
- "I'm wasting precious work time!"
- "But (child, spouse, etc.) needs me."
- "I'm doing something wrong."
- "I don't deserve this."
- "I'd better hurry up and get back to…"
- "I'm being too selfish."
- "I'm taking too much time away from what I 'should' be doing."

Recognize that these thoughts are common and natural. They arise from the conditions and patterns of your life thus far. However, they are just thoughts and not necessarily true. You can note "thinking" when these thoughts arise, and then return to your intention of self-care. You are entering into a new way of being, and will need to re-pattern your habits around this. Let yourself notice how it feels when you are really taking care of yourself, and notice the effect this way of being has on your moods, energy and relationships. Self-care and quietude are not optional luxuries to take advantage of if you somehow "find" the time. These are essential in order for you to achieve complete balance, and therefore health, and it is important to clear the space for these nourishing rituals in your life.

The choice of activities and how many you incorporate into your cleanse is up to you. If making time for self-care feels difficult or overwhelming, start with one or two practices that feel the most attainable to you, and schedule them in. This might mean one massage and two yoga or guided meditation classes during your 14-day cleanse. It might mean going to bed 30 minutes early each night and scheduling two baths during your cleansing weeks. What feels most relaxing, attainable and healing to you?

> *Practice letting go, surrendering and trusting in the natural flow of things.*
> ❀
> *Remember that you have time for everything that is in divine right alignment.*

Even by scheduling less, you will be practicing self-care as you will have more time to do the things you normally do without having to rush. Allow time to stop and notice the world around you through the senses, be in your daily experience, and move more slowly. Do you tend to over-schedule? Avoid scheduling clients during your lunch-time or scheduling early morning activities that encroach on your breakfast. If you do not have flexibility in your schedule, enter each day and each task mindfully, calmly and centered, then add relaxing therapies during your evenings, weekends or days off.

Ask for help from those around you, whether at home or at work. Who do you know that could take on cooking a meal for your children, running an errand or cleaning the bathroom? Make requests.

Release some of your to-do list. The more practice you get at this, the easier it becomes. At first it may seem impossible — *everything* needs to get done, now! If this is the case, do a one-minute deep breathing meditation, then return calm and centered to your list.

Ask yourself:
1. What tasks or projects can be simplified so that they take less time or stress?
2. What tasks or projects can get pushed back a day, a couple days or until next week to lighten my load?
3. What tasks or projects can I delegate to someone else?
4. What tasks or projects are really not important and I can let go of entirely?

Making the Cleanse Yours

A beautiful foundation of Ayurveda is the concept of treating the individual. Ayurveda understands that we are all a unique expression of the universal qualities in all of nature. In line with this, there will be opportunities to adjust and make room for doing this cleanse to fit your constitutional tendencies, the state you are in, and your comfort level. A guiding principle throughout is to listen to yourself and the wisdom of your body and mind. You can make the cleanse more gentle at any time by scaling back on the ghee intake and/or herbal supplements. For more ideas on how to individualize your cleanse according to your unique body type, complete the mindbody self-assessment in Chapter 2, and review the suggestions for each constitutional type on pages 101 - 102.

THE MINI CLEANSE

There are times when you feel like you need to clean up your body and mind but just don't have the space and energy to do the full home cleanse. In this case, the mini cleanse is a great, short clean-up you can do in one week to get you started on making this an annual or bi-annual habit.

Traditionally, panchakarma cleansing was used to help the body transition into each new season and was done regularly at seasonal changes as part of a preventative healthcare regimen. While doing the whole two week program two to four times per year may feel daunting, this shorter, more mellow cleanse can be a great alternative in between your annual or bi-annual

full cleanse. Additionally, the protocol for the two week cleanse may be a big departure from your usual diet. In this case, starting with this mini cleanse may be a great first step or "warm up" to the full Mindbody Cleanse. And, finally, employing the mini cleanse when feeling under the weather or just "junked out" is a great way to change things around and support the mindbody. Whatever the reason, this short cleanse can still offer a boost in energy and metabolic efficiency.

The basic rhythm to remember for this one week mini cleanse is 2-3-2. In this shortened version, the Preparation Phase lasts two days, the Purification Phase lasts three days and the Rebuilding Phase, two days. Follow the diet guidelines for these phases just as described in the full program. You will also add the lemon-ginger slices or lemon digestive tonic to your diet on the last two days. However, in this mellower version, you do not take the ghee in the mornings. You do not do the purgation or enema. We recommend you take triphala for the whole week, and at least one week following the mini cleanse. Triphala should be taken with a cup of warm water. The recommended does is 1-2 capsules about an hour before bedtime and 1-2 capsules in the morning before breakfast.

To summarize:

- Two days of eating a simple easy-to-digest whole foods diet without heavy meat, dairy, oils, nuts, sugar, alcohol, caffeine or gluten
- Three days of a primarily split mung diet, augmented with cooked veggies and minimal amounts of cooked non-gluten grains

- Two days back to the simple preparation diet, adding in the Ginger Lemon Appetizer (page 239) before meals.
- Throughout the whole week and at least one week afterwards, take triphala.
- Drink lots of warm to hot water and digestive teas throughout the day.
- Eat plenty of beets and green veggies throughout the week.
- Exercise a little each day.
- Practice balancing the nervous system through meditation, yoga, pranayama, relaxation, baths, etc.

As with the full program, notice your relationship to food and eating and notice how you feel. Acknowledging these cause-and-effect patterns offers you information that leads to more skillful and wise living.

ENHANCEMENTS

Stronger Digestive Reset Protocol
If you need additional digestive support, this alternative protocol can give you a greater boost. This differs from the regular digestive reset protocol in that you will be taking increasing quantities of digestive support for three days, along with the Lemon Digestive Tonic, before meals. If you are adding digestive supplements (such as trikatu, Cool Digest, Pitta Digest, Warm Digest, etc.) to your cleanse, take these in increasing quantities. If not, take the Ginger Lemon Appetizer slices (page 239) in increasing quantities, as tolerated (they can get spicy!). Optionally, you can take all three before meals: Lemon Digestive Tonic, increasing quantities of digestive supplements and a ginger-lemon slice.

Day 1 Rebuilding
- Go back to the Preparation Phase diet for at least three days: low fat, lots of veggies, and no oils/gluten/dairy/sugar/red meat or other hard to digest foods. Include plenty of fresh vegetables in your diet and have green smoothies and juices as much as possible. Continue eating the grated beet salad if you are enjoying it.
- Take 2 ginger-lemon slices and/or digestive supplements before each meal.
- Introduce *small* amounts of probiotics into your diet. Good sources are: a probiotic supplement, sauerkraut or kim chi or other *live* fermented foods, such as miso, blue green algae, and tempeh.
- Take Lemon Digestive Tonic before meals (recipe on page 150).

Day 2 Rebuilding
- Continue taking the lemon water before your meals.
- Increase to 3 ginger-lemon slices and/or digestive supplements before each meal.
- Continue including probiotics into your diet.
- Continue with Preparation Phase diet.

Day 3 Rebuilding
- Continue taking the lemon water before your meals.
- Increase to 4 ginger-lemon slices and/or digestive supplements before each meal.
- Continue with Preparation Phase diet.

Following the third day of the Rebuilding Phase, you can continue to take as much digestive support as needed. Be careful not to create too much fire – if you begin to feel heartburn, acid reflux or other hot conditions, you can ease back or eliminate these altogether. If you are eliminating normally for your body type (see page 115) and food moves through the digestive tract (rather than just sitting heavily in your stomach) and you are hungry at regular mealtimes, these are signs that digestion is working well.

Additional Bastis (enemas)

For dry constipation, you can do a longer series of bastis as follows:

Day 1 Post-Cleanse – Administer a decoction basti:

* Boil 1 Tbsp dashamula in 2 cups of water. Simmer with lid off for 5-10 minutes. (If you do not have dashamula, you can use plain water.)
* Cool to body temperature.
* Strain and add ½ cup warm sesame oil and use for basti.
* Retain the liquid as long as you comfortably can.

Day 2 Post-Cleanse – Take an oil basti:

* Heat 1 cup sesame oil to body temp.
* Administer basti and retain as long as you comfortably can.
* Do not eat for at least 2 hours after.

Subsequent Enemas – You can take bastis for several days in a row (up to 7 days) for conditions of extremely dry stools or constipation. Alternate between the decoction and the oil enemas, always ending the series with an oil enema.

Nasya

Nasya is an herbal oil that is administered through the nasal passages to lubricate and nourish the tissues. It protects the sensitive tissue of the nose and sinuses and is a deterrent for irritants and allergens. Traditionally, nasya is used in panchakarma and can be added to your home PK version. Place 2-5 drops in each nostril first thing in the morning, while lying on your back. Take several deep breaths through the nose.

Tikta Grita - Herbal Ghee

This is a traditional ghee made with several herbs. This ghee can be taken during the purification phase instead of regular ghee. The overall quality of this formula is very bitter and is especially helpful in detoxifying the liver. If you have difficulty digesting fats, this can be helpful in digesting the ghee. However, because of its very bitter quality, it can increase vata and be aggravating to those with a strong vata tendency.

Chapter 4
Working With Our Indulgences

"When I am hungry I seek nourishment and when I feel gnawing unrest or other painful emotions I seek the changes in my life which will resolve the unhealthy and painful feelings."

– Bernie Siegel

If you are dealing with any addiction issues, it is valuable to take these into consideration as you are preparing for your cleanse. Addictions may prolong your Preparation Phase, and that's okay. Be kind to yourself and take the time you need. However, beware of using an addiction as an excuse to never get around to cleansing. Do the best you can and start your cleanse anyway. As your body moves more and more into balance, your addictions will likely become easier to address.

Along with the opportunity to examine your relationship to food in general during this cleanse comes the opportunity to evaluate your relationship to specific foods and substances that can cause a stronger and possibly addictive reaction, such as caffeine, alcohol, tobacco and sugar. Most of these are socially accepted and many people don't think twice when consuming them daily, or even several times per day. All of these substances offer some mind-altering side effects that make it easy to come to rely on them: they get us up in the morning, put us to sleep at night or strengthen our focus and concentration. Once reliance is built up, the removal of these substances can result in "withdrawal symptoms." In this section, we will cover how to deal with or lessen these symptoms to make your cleansing experience more comfortable. You will find that as you lessen reliance on the qualities these substances offer you, your body will naturally return to its cycles of waking and resting in harmony with the cycles of nature and, as your body moves closer to balance, energy and mental clarity will become better than ever.

It is important to note that the occasional use of any substance is not a cause for concern. Of course you will enjoy a slice of pumpkin pie at a holiday meal, or share a glass of wine with a partner or friend once in a while. Ayurveda even recommends smoking herbal cigarettes for certain conditions as a therapeutic treatment, and coffee can be used in the treatment of asthma. Green tea contains many beneficial properties such as antioxidants and amino acids, even though it contains small amounts of caffeine. *This section is aimed at addressing the reliance on these substances for daily functioning.* If you regularly use any of these substances to wake you up, get focused, calm you down, or any other purpose other than to nourish your being, this is a wonderful opportunity to release dependency on it and begin to cultivate a healthy relationship to it.

Key Nutrients in Detoxification
When removing addictive substances, good nutrition can make your experience more easeful. In modern studies on addiction and detoxification, several key nutrients have been identified that can lessen withdrawal symptoms and speed up the body's detoxification process. The chart on the following page outlines these nutrients and offers suggestions of whole food sources that provide them. These are foods that are recommended during your Preparation and Rebuilding Phases. If you are choosing well-balanced meals during this time, you are likely getting ideal nutrition for detoxification.

Key Nutrients in Detoxification - Whole Food Sources

B Vitamins

Oatmeal	Fortified tofu
Rice	Lentils
Bananas	Avocado
Dark leafy greens	Sweet potato
Potatoes	Broccoli

Vitamin C

Bell peppers	Berries
Dark leafy greens	Citrus fruits
Kiwis	Tomatoes
Broccoli	Peas
Cauliflower	Papayas
Brussels sprouts	Pineapples

Calcium

Dark leafy greens	Black eyed peas
Broccoli	Fortified tofu
Quinoa	Sesame seeds
White beans	Seaweed
Dried figs	

Key Nutrients in Detoxification - Whole Food Sources

Magnesium

Pumpkin seeds	Millet
Dark leafy greens	White beans
Soybeans	Kidney beans
Brown rice	Lentils
Quinoa	Avocados

Chromium

Broccoli	Potatoes
Mushrooms	Bananas
Asparagus	Prunes
Whole grains	Black pepper
Green beans	Thyme

Glutamine

Lentils	Carrots
Split peas	Brussels sprouts
Beans (esp. soy)	Quinoa
Spinach	Millet
Kale	Brown rice
Parsley	Pumpkin seeds
Beets	Sunflower seeds

Addiction and Constitution

Addictive tendencies, and the ability to gracefully remove addictive substances, are sometimes predicted by constitution. Notice if you resonate with any of the tendencies associated with your prakruti, but remember that this is not always true. Use this information only to better understand your tendencies rather than embracing them because it is "supposed" to be true for your particular constitution.

Vata-dominant people tend to be able to give up addictions for short periods of time but tend to return to them, or to switch to a different addiction. Vatas are strongly affected by addictive substances, because of their tendency toward heightened sensitivity.

Pitta-dominant people tend to have very strong will power and can give up just about anything if they put their mind to it. The key here is for the individual to choose to give it up, rather than being told they must give it up. Personal choice is very important to pittas.

Kapha-dominant people tend to have a greater ability to remain healthy despite bad habits because of their strong constitution. However, they also tend to have the most difficulty giving them up, in keeping with their tendency toward attachment when out of balance.

CAFFEINE

Caffeine is one of the most used and most socially accepted mind/energy-altering substances. The withdrawal symptoms of caffeine are well known: headaches, fatigue, lethargy, difficulty concentrating, difficulty "getting going" in the morning (both energy levels and bowels), irritability and cravings for emergency food, such as sugar. Despite the side effects of removing it, this is a far better choice than continuing to use caffeine once you learn the long term effects of habitual use. These include:

- Anxiety and panic attacks
- Insomnia
- Weakened adrenal function
- Weakened central nervous system
- Increased blood pressure
- Increased serum cholesterol
- Chronic fatigue, muscle fatigue
- Increased heart rate
- Dehydration
- Lowered blood sugar, causing sugar cravings
- Osteoporosis due to reduced absorption of calcium
- Anemia due to reduced absorption of iron
- Heart arrhythmia, tachycardia and palpitations
- Fibrocystic breast disease
- Kidney stones
- Prostate enlargement
- Loss of bladder control
- Ulcers and gastritis

One of the best tips we can give regarding weaning caffeine is that the slower you taper your consumption, the easier the transition will be. For someone who regularly drinks 2-3 cups of coffee per day, you might follow a two-week schedule similar to the following:

- **Days 1-3**: Drink black tea in the morning, have 1 cup of coffee after lunch, on a full stomach.
- **Days 4-6**: Drink green tea in the morning, have 1 cup of black tea after lunch, on a full stomach.
- **Days 7-9**: Drink only green tea but allow yourself 2-4 cups per day.
- **Days 10-12**: Cut down to 1-2 cups of green tea per day.
- Cut down by ½ - 1 cup per day each day until you feel you can go without it.

Of course, tailor this to your needs, consistently decreasing the amount of caffeine you are taking in. It is best to wean yourself from caffeine before you begin your cleanse to avoid caffeine withdrawal at the same time that you may be feeling some cleansing symptoms. However, beware of using this excuse to never get to the cleansing phase. If you are having difficulty cutting out caffeine after trying

❀❀❀❀❀❀❀❀❀❀❀❀❀❀❀

❀ *Adrian's Experience:* ❀
❀ *"I once had a cleanse group participant* ❀
❀ *who brewed a cup of coffee several times* ❀
❀ *during her cleanse, only to hold it in her* ❀
❀ *hands and smell it, then dump it all out!* ❀
❀ *Sometimes the ritual of making the coffee* ❀
❀ *can be as powerful as drinking it."* ❀

❀❀❀❀❀❀❀❀❀❀❀❀❀❀❀

several of the tactics that follow, just start your cleanse and do your best. Choose green tea, rather than coffee. Even decaf coffee is very acidic and dehydrating, so it is not a good choice during your cleanse.

Tips for gracefully removing caffeine from your diet include:
- Drink plenty of water (more than usual) as headaches are often the result of dehydration caused by caffeine.
- Get plenty of rest and reduce stress.
- Also cut out sugar, as these two substances tend to perpetuate one another.
- Support your adrenals with adaptogenic herbs. Tulsi, in capsule or tea form, is an excellent tonic for the adrenals and is gentle enough to take before a cleanse. Ginseng is helpful, as it nourishes the adrenals and also gives an energy boost. Licorice is an excellent adrenal tonic as well. For a nice caffeine removal tea, combine licorice, tulsi, and ginger. Ashwaganda, rhodiola and astragalus are other helpful adaptogenic herbs. As these are a little heavier, they are better for after a cleanse, but are certainly a better choice than coffee during the Preparation and Purification Phases.
- Increase intake of vitamins B and C, potassium, magnesium, calcium, zinc and iron.
- Potassium bicarbonate tablets will make the body more alkaline and help decrease withdrawal symptoms.
- Dashamula is a natural pain reliever and may be used in place of acetaminophen or ibuprofen for headaches. Make a strong tea

from the dashamula root by combining 2 Tbsp dashamula powder in 2 cups water in a medium pot. Bring to a boil, lower heat and simmer until liquid is reduced by half. Take ¼ cup; store remaining tea in the refrigerator and reheat before taking.

- Suck on cardamom pods. This has a similar taste as coffee and antidotes the effect of caffeine.
- Drink dandelion or nettle tea to replace coffee, replenish minerals and support the liver.
- Place a cool ice cloth on your forehead and put heat on your feet for 20-30 minutes to alleviate headaches.
- If you feel you cannot get coffee out of your diet, at least limit yourself to one cup on a full stomach and brew it with a pinch of cardamom - these measures will help protect the lining of the stomach from the acidic nature of coffee. Be sure to drink a large glass of water before and after, as coffee is also very dehydrating.
- If you need more energy, try adding blue-green algae during the Preparation Phase.
- If what you need is something hot and dark to drink in the morning, try replacing coffee with a tea substitute. Dandelion root and chicory root make great teas that are rich and dark. There are also plenty of "herbal coffee" substitutes on the market. LeRoux's instant chicory is a good choice, as it has only one ingredient (chicory). Inka, Pero, Cafix, Tecchino and other brands are available in various combinations of herbs, but check labels for added sugar. Also, it is best to find an herbal coffee substitute that doesn't include barley, as it is recommended to avoid gluten-containing products during the cleanse.

ALCOHOL

Alcohol is another highly accepted substance that has addictive properties. Regular alcohol consumption is linked to hypoglycemia (low blood sugar) and sugar addiction. Studies have shown that the brains of alcoholics are insulin resistant, meaning they are losing their ability to utilize glucose (sugar) for fuel. The acetic acid that alcohol provides can be used for fuel when insulin resistance is present. For this reason, the brain soon needs alcohol to keep brain cells alive. Modern research has found, however, that when insulin resistance of the brain occurs, fat can still be used when sugar is no longer an option. (See bibliography for more on this.) Because we are resetting our bodies to utilize fat as a source of fuel, this cleanse is excellent for helping to detox from alcohol. The daily ghee during main cleanse will be key.

If you have difficulty giving up alcohol, this is a sign of addiction, and all the more reason to take some time off. Alcohol increases the fire element in the body, leading to excess acid (consider the term "fire water"). Alcohol also produces a toxic metabolite called acetaldehyde, which causes damage to the brain, nerves and liver tissue, as well as poisoning the bloodstream. According to the Ayurvedic view, it has a numbing effect, making the mind dull and lethargic, which is referred to as a *tamasic* mind state.

Some tips for easing the removal of alcohol:

- Follow the suggestions for removing sugar as outlined in this chapter, as alcohol addiction is often a form of sugar addiction.
- Cut out caffeine. Often we end up on the roller coaster, needing substances to get us going in the morning and through the day (coffee, chocolate, sugar) and then a sedative to help us sleep at night (alcohol, marijuana). By removing these other substances, you are allowing your body the opportunity to tune in to its natural rhythms.
- If you normally drink alcohol for its sedative and calming effects, consider drinking chamomile or tulsi tea. These are both very calming while nourishing your adrenals. Other nervines that may be helpful are passionflower, skullcap, kava kava and hops. While these can be very heavy to take before a cleanse, they are a better choice than alcohol.
- Spend time relaxing, away from technology.
- Find other non-alcoholic beverages you enjoy. Try combining cranberry juice, sparkling water and a splash of apple juice for a fun drink to have at parties.
- Bitters (such as Swedish bitters in supplement form) and bitter foods (such as kale, spinach, chard) are helpful for supporting the liver and fighting sugar cravings.

TOBACCO

Cigarettes today contain far more than just tobacco – most contain several hundred cancer-causing chemicals including dioxins, which also causes genetic mutations and brain damage. It is widely known that smoking cigarettes causes lung and liver cancer. With so many strikes against it, why is it so hard to quit? Because of the "benefits:" tobacco balances the nervous system, which calms anxiety and stimulates brain function. Tobacco offers calm emotions and the ability to think clearly. We have seen many people attempt to quit, only to go back to it during a stressful day at work. Because the dependency is focused on calming the nerves, many of the suggestions for cutting out alcohol apply here as well. The cleansing diet we outline in this book is very helpful in and of itself to aid in quitting smoking.

Other tips to make quitting easier include:

- Decide on a clear plan of action ahead of time. Write it down. Share the plan with someone that will support you in the process. To go "cold turkey" or to wean off slowly is the first decision to make. Then go from there. Choose a date (or dates) and put it on your calendar where you will see it.
- Get clear on why you want to quit. What is it costing you? What do you see happening in five years if you don't quit? Ten years? Twenty years? Write these down – you might want to refer back to them.
- Reduce or eliminate excess stress, since this is most often when cravings strike. During this cleanse, we recommend taking time away from social activity as much as possible and scheduling in relaxing activities instead, such as a professional massage, saunas and baths. All of these are

helpful when quitting smoking.

- Include yoga and other forms of exercise into your routine. Yoga is especially beneficial because it helps the mind and body deal with stress in a healthy way, but all forms of gentle exercise are great.
- Try the pranayama breathing techniques outlined in Chapter 5. These can help tremendously when a craving hits and will calm the central nervous system in a much more nourishing way.
- Notice habits around smoking and replace these with new, positive habits, such as exercise, drinking water or a hobby you enjoy.
- Re-pattern habits by varying your routine from what you normally do and stay away from places you would normally smoke.
- Spend time with non-smoking friends.
- Add teas made from calming herbs and herbs that are high in minerals, such as tulsi, chamomile, valerian, red clover leaf, alfalfa and mullein leaf.
- Add triphala to your cleanse. Because it is high in vitamin C, it will help to remove the nicotine from your body more quickly, thus lessening withdrawal symptoms.
- Ginseng and ashwaganda both help the mindbody respond to stress in a more healthy way. These are stronger herbs than chamomile and tulsi, and are "heavier," thus not as ideal for the Preparation Phase (very good for the Rejuvenation Phase) but are a much better alternative to smoking!
- Surround yourself with positive people and choose positive affirmations to use. Make your affirmations simple enough that you can remember them when a tough moment arises, and/or write them

down and place them where you will see them often. Ideas are, "I choose health and freedom from addictions," or "I am creating a new, healthy, smoke-free life," then, "I successfully quit smoking and I am healthier because of it," or "I love and respect my body. I am no longer a smoker."

SUGAR

In a culture where sugar is abundant and cheap, this is a substance that has become vastly over-used. Sugar consumption has skyrocketed over the past 200 years: in 1800 the average person consumed 18 pounds of sugar per person per year. Today, that number is up to 150 pounds per person per year. Consumption is greater among children, indicating that this number will only continue to rise if we don't make some major dietary changes.

Some researchers say sugar is more addictive than cocaine, so it is not a surprise that sugar cravings are one of the most common struggles we have helped people deal with. Over-consumption of sugar is linked to insulin resistance, Type II diabetes, weight gain, obesity, mood swings, tooth decay, nutritional deficiencies, hypoglycemia (low blood sugar), inflammation, anxiety and depression, bloating and gas, and Candida yeast overgrowth (which has its own long list of problems, such as chronic ear, sinus and yeast infections and chronic fatigue). While many people frown upon tobacco and alcohol consumption, the dangers and addictive nature of sugar is rarely a consideration by most.

The sweet taste is associated with love and nurturing from the time we are born. Mother's milk is sweet in taste and high in the milk sugar lactose. It is common in our culture to give children sweets as a reward for being "good" and to show our affection. Cake and ice cream are used to celebrate special occasions, which end up happening so often that it isn't a "special" food anymore. Weekly or even daily we are celebrating a birthday, retirement, secular or religious holiday, promotion, baby shower, new birth, grand opening...the list goes on. Of course, this is not to say that you shouldn't enjoy a slice of birthday cake on your birthday, but it is important to become mindful of how often, how much and for what reasons you are consuming it. From this place, you can begin to cultivate a healthy relationship to it in which you are choosing it, rather than eating it daily due to uncontrollable cravings.

Sugar is hard to avoid, since it is in 80% of the products on grocery store shelves. Besides the obvious culprits of cookies, pastries, soda and cakes, it is found in almost all salad dressings, ketchup, processed meats, nut butters, canned fruits and vegetables, crackers, soups, yogurt and jams. Once you start paying attention to sugar and reading labels, ask yourself – When was the last time you went just one day without eating something with sugar in it? Likely, your answer will be months, or even years. If we aren't snacking on some dark chocolate after a meal ("But it's got antioxidants!"), we are consuming it unknowingly in ketchup or almond butter. The best way to avoid these hidden sources of sugar is to choose fresh, whole foods and prepare them yourself at home. This is exactly what we are doing during this cleanse

through a simplified, nourishing diet.

When removing sugar from the diet for the cleanse, some initial symptoms of withdrawal are common – usually in the form of sugar cravings. Sometimes getting to the bottom of your sugar cravings can help make the removal process easier. Cravings for sugar are often the result of two common conditions: blood sugar fluctuations and Candida overgrowth.

Blood Sugar Imbalances
Most Americans have lost the ability to properly regulate blood sugar. This is primarily due to poor diet and lifestyle habits. A diet high in refined carbohydrates and sugars, alcohol, caffeine, and tobacco lead to problems with the endocrine system - particularly the liver, thyroid, pancreas, and adrenals. Continuous high stress levels also contribute to blood sugar problems. How do you know if your sugar cravings are the result of blood sugar fluctuations? One of the first signs that blood sugar regulation is going haywire is daily drops in blood sugar levels.

Signs of low blood sugar (hypoglycemia) include:
- Headaches
- Fatigue
- Feeling light-headed/dizzy
- Inability to concentrate
- Irritability, mood swings
- Depression, anxiety
- Nervousness
- Heart palpitations
- Blurred vision
- Confusion
- Cravings for sweets

- Fainting
- Night sweats
- Weakness in the legs
- Constant hunger
- Cold hands or feet
- Muscle twitches or cramps
- Restlessness
- Anti-social behavior

Being aware of these symptoms is extremely important because they are the first warning signs of much more serious problems, particularly Type II diabetes. Though it may initially seem counterintuitive, low blood sugar can lead to high blood sugar.

The normal functioning of blood sugar regulation goes like this: when you eat, your body transforms that food into glucose, which we use as fuel. The pancreas has the job of releasing insulin, which allows the right amount of glucose to be used for fuel now, and sending the rest to the liver, to be stored for use later. When all of the glucose in the blood stream is used up, the liver receives a message to release some of its stores, therefore keeping blood sugar levels in check. When our bodies are functioning optimally, there is very little fluctuation happening.

Initial fluctuations are usually linked to an over active pancreas, in which it secretes more insulin than is needed. The pancreas isn't functioning properly because of exhaustion – usually the result of "grazing" (snacking all day) or a diet rich in high glycemic foods, such as white sugar and white flour, that cause a sharp spike in blood sugar levels and, in turn, a spike

in release of insulin. Both of these scenarios ask the pancreas to work double time.

When there is excess insulin in the blood stream, the liver never gets the message to release stored glucose, and so blood sugar levels stay low. Because the body is not regulating blood sugar levels on its own, we need to eat more to keep them up. When you are having a sugar craving, this is your body asking for more fuel, because sugar is the food that can most quickly be converted into energy. While resorting to "emergency" foods, like white flour and white sugar, may help the symptoms at the time, it is making the problem worse in the long run by further stressing the pancreas.

Because the liver is holding on to all of its stores instead of releasing them as it should, it eventually gets full. Once the liver and cells have stored all the glycogen they can hold, the excess glucose is directed to fat cells for storage, hence the weight gain that is associated with pre-diabetes, particularly around the stomach. Further, when the liver and cells are full they eventually stop responding to insulin. This is called insulin resistance: the cells are not responding to insulin, or need excessive amounts in order to stimulate a response. Eventually, more and more insulin is needed, and soon the pancreas is totally exhausted. Once the pancreas cannot produce enough insulin, blood sugar levels remain high and the result is Type II diabetes.

Candida Overgrowth
The other common cause of sugar cravings is Candida yeast overgrowth. *Candida albicans*

is a naturally occurring yeast organism that is found in the digestive tract in small quantities. However, this particular organism can become over grown from a diet high in refined sugars or alcohol, after taking antibiotics that wipe out the good bacteria that normally keep the bad bacteria in check, or when then there is a change in hormone levels, such during as pregnancy or menopause.

When Candida albicans is overgrown, one of the major symptoms is strong cravings for sugar, bread or alcohol. Adding probiotic-rich foods to the diet, cleansing seasonally, limiting sugar intake and working to build strong digestive fire and immunity are all key in healing from Candida. This cleanse covers all of these areas, so if you are dealing with a yeast overgrowth condition, this cleansing program may be very helpful. Ayurvedic herbs that discourage the further growth of Candida yeast include turmeric, which we use quite a lot of in this cleanse, tulsi (also known as holy basil, very nice as a tea throughout the cleanse), asafeotida, neem, cloves, nutmeg and cardamom.

When dealing with blood sugar fluctuations, Candida or just plain sugar addiction, eliminating sugar can be difficult. However, from extensive personal experience with all of these conditions, we can assure you that the first three days without sugar are the hardest.

Some tips to ease the removal of sugar are:
- Add gymnema sylvestre to your cleanse. We have had clients (even when not cleansing) add this herb to their daily routine and rave about how their sugar cravings have completely disappeared! More information on this is found in the Herbs section in Chapter 7.
- Avoid low blood sugar crashes by building meals wisely during the Preparation and Rebuilding Phases: be sure to include plenty of fiber (legumes, vegetables, fruit, whole grains), clean protein (legumes, lean chicken or turkey, seeds) and healthy fats (avocados, seeds) in your meals. These slow the absorption of glucose into the bloodstream, making fuel last longer – ideally until the next meal.
- Check labels. There are about 100 different names for different kinds of sugars and artificial sweeteners (which are worse than sugar). As a general rule during this cleanse, if you don't understand an ingredient on a package, don't eat it.
- Drink plenty of water.
- End your meal with a bitter bite. Not only does this curb sweet cravings at the end of a meal, it also begins to re-pattern old habits.
- Sometimes sweet cravings are the result of too much or not enough protein intake. Consider how much protein you are getting and decide if an adjustment would be beneficial. To determine how much protein is right for you, multiply your body weight by 0.36; the result is the number grams of protein you should be taking in each day. This, of course, is an estimate, as time of life, prakruti, vikruti, lifestyle, exercise levels and stress levels can alter the amount of protein you may need.
- Satisfy sweet cravings in a healthy way by

including naturally sweet foods into your diet, such as fresh fruit, yams, sweet potatoes, carrots and beets.

- Eat fruit at the beginning of a meal or by themselves. Ayurveda teaches us that sweet foods digest fastest. When eating these after slower digesting foods, they will begin to ferment in the digestive tract, further exacerbating Candida overgrowth conditions and causing gas and bloating. Sweet foods also stimulate the appetite; so eating them at the beginning of a meal is beneficial.
- Add a small amount of live sauerkraut or other probiotic-rich foods to meals. While this is too strong of a food for the Preparation or Purification Phases, it is very beneficial during the Rebuilding Phase, when we are working to repopulate the beneficial bacteria in the gut. Adding a probiotic supplement is also beneficial during this time.
- Test blood sugar levels at home using a glucometer.
- Emotional attachments may be equally as difficult as physiological addiction when it comes to sugar.
- Vitamins B and C, chromium, calcium, magnesium and glutamine are beneficial to keep blood sugar levels even. All of these nutrients are also extremely helpful when removing any addiction from the body and speeding up recovery time, as listed in the beginning of this section.

FOOD ADDICTION

This cleanse can be a major contributor to overcoming food addiction. Because we are simplifying the diet and learning to relate to our food in terms of nourishment, rather than entertainment, this is a perfect opportunity to consider all ways and reasons for which you have been using food. Notice the other uses you have for food, beyond simply fueling your mindbody: comfort, anxiety, boredom, anger, resentment, avoiding emotions, happiness, celebration, connecting with others, distraction. Notice how these are false. Notice how these stop you short from fully living life and fully experiencing each moment.

A great place to start with unwinding food addiction is to identify your emotions or reasons for using food. From there, you can think of ways to deal with that particular emotion or situation rather than using food. The chart on the following page address some common misplaced uses for food with some starting points for dealing with them. If one or some of these resonate with you, take them on as your own and explore how you can shift your way of being in relation to these situations.

WHAT ARE YOU USING FOOD FOR?

(Try this instead.)

Comfort

Stay warm
Wear comfortable clothing
Choose simple and warming foods

Anxiety

Pranayama breathing techniques
Meditation
Exercise
Laughter

Boredom

Find work that you love
Take on a hobby
Meditation
Laughter

Anger

Exercise
Non-violent communication
Journaling
Practice surrender
Rose essential oil
Drink plenty of water
"Cool off" by swimming in cool water and
eating cooling foods

Happiness

Hugging
Body movement/exercise/dancing
Journaling
Giving gratitude through words, letters, gifts

Celebration

Practice ritual
Journaling
Body Movement/exercise/dancing
Attending a special event (theatre, music, etc.)

*Connection/
Belonging*

Re-pattern thoughts about belonging with
affirmations and positive self-talk
Hugging
Practice listening
Holding hands
Meditation
Pranayama breathing techniques

Another excellent resource on the
issue of emotional eating is Geneen
Roth. Her book *Women, Food and
God* is recommended reading for
anyone dealing with food addiction.

Chapter 5
Stress Management

"To be enlightened is to be without anxiety of imperfections."

– Zen Master Seung Sahn

Stress management and self-care practices are just as important as diet and herbs in supporting a successful cleanse. Try to do some stress management and self-care practices every day. Remember, this cleanse draws from traditional PK, where participants are on residential retreat. Ease in the mind and body are essential to facilitate the release of stored emotions and toxins.

Yoga, meditation, pranayama (breath work) and relaxation are the most important stress-management practices to include in your cleanse. We recommend incorporating these daily practices as much as possible so that you have a consistent way to check in with yourself during the cleanse, as well as practices in place to help reduce stress. We want to be mindful and aware of what is happening but, even with our best intentions, it is so easy to forget. A lot. This is because we are not practiced in being mindful. We are used to our minds running amok — fantasizing, planning, reviewing, judging, craving — in a vague haze, all of which we may not even recognize until we start becoming aware. So, what helps us remember? Practice. There is probably no getting around it, we need to practice to reconfigure the neural pathways into ones of noticing and paying attention to what is occurring in the moment. We will introduce you to some simple do-able practices in this book. You may grow to love them!

YOGA FOR CLEANSING

We recommend yoga as a stress management practice in this program because yoga and Ayurveda have a long history of inter-enhancing ideals and practices. However, if yoga just doesn't speak to you, find another physical practice that energizes the body while simultaneously calming the mind. It is important to have some kind of meditative movement as a practice, be it qigong, yoga, tai chi or some other form, that enables our connection to the physical experience as it is happening. When we are aware of our body, it short-circuits the scattered, over-busy mind. The body is only present in the moment. It is not the body of 10 years ago or even 10 minutes ago and it is not the body of the future. When you tune into your body, it immediately brings you into the present moment. As you focus on the sense experience of the body, the mind becomes stable and more focused. In addition, within the practice itself, we learn to be with what is, without reacting. For example, we learn to take a full and deep breath with a relaxed restorative pose as well as with a challenging, intense pose. The movement is organized with the breath in a manner that is conducive to creating a full, more complete breath. This alone triggers a parasympathetic response. Additionally, the coordination of the breath with movement gives the mind a consistent anchor that we can rest our attention on. This consistency creates continuity and a meditative state of mind.

Yoga As Stability

Yoga can help create stable ground to support you as you move through the detoxification process. As toxins and stored emotions begin to disentangle and move through the body, the steady, mindful practice of yoga can help you to be with any difficult emotions and changes in the body, without getting caught up in their stories. Yoga creates a stable ground of support during the cleanse. We do this by setting an even rhythm to the practice, established by an even breath—meaning the inhale and exhale last approximately the same time. We can also create stability in the practice by keeping this rhythm as we flow into and out of poses. In general, the practice should be slow, deliberate and even. Try holding poses a little longer than you would normally, and move slowly between them. Pay close attention to the feet and hips to help ground the practice in the stability of the earth element.

Yoga and the Digestive System
Additionally, the practice itself enhances the cleansing effects. During the cleanse, we are moving toxins from the deep tissues into the digestive system to be metabolized or ejected. To facilitate this process, the many channels of the body need to be open and unobstructed. Yoga enhances this cleansing method because the shape created by each pose, combined with deep breathing, leads to openings in the body and channels. This supports the movement of prana, or life energy, throughout the body.

To facilitate this, we focus on opening the digestive system in particular. The digestive organs lie under the rib cage on both sides of the body, and into the whole belly area parallel to the front of the hip bones. In the back of the body, the kidneys lie just below the rib cage. So, focusing on the lower half of the torso is a key element in yoga practice for this cleanse. This can be achieved by movement that opens the area under the rib cage on the inhale, and closes and contracts this area on the exhale. This creates a stretching and squeezing effect on the digestive organs. Twisting movements squeeze the digestive organs and, as you release these poses, blood flows directly back into them. This creates a nourishing effect on the organs of digestion. When the digestive organs are stimulated, we have greater capacity to digest the toxins that have been dislodged. The organs have three dimensions in the body, so we must move and stretch this area three ways: front to back, side-to-side and twisting the torso.

To summarize, a cleansing yoga practice should have two main focal points:
- A calm, grounded quality
- A focus on the digestive area of the body

The following pages offer some sample yoga practices to achieve this. Videos of these practices are also available at meadowheartayurveda.com.

Always open your practice by sitting mindfully. You can do a pranayama practice or a short meditation. See pages 75 - 78 for this, then, try moving into one of the two cleansing practices that follow.

Yoga for Cleansing Sequences

"We establish a calm, abiding center, not to fortify ourselves against the chaos of life, but to help us become resilient, tolerant, and accepting of the inevitable, perplexing, and often agonizing losses we all go through. A calm, abiding center and a fully engaged life, therefore, go hand in hand. This inner tempering through the fire of practice allows us to live at higher and higher levels of charge: to feel intensely, love intensely and work intensely without fracturing in the process."

– Donna Farhi

Yoga for Cleansing
Short Practice, 30-40 minutes
For an even shorter, 10–20 minute practice, do postures 1–10, and then end with shavasana.

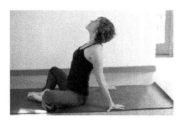

1. **Cobbler** *(badha konasana)* with chest opening. On an inhale, lean back into your hands and open the rib cage, letting the lungs fully open.

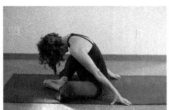

2. **On your exhale,** let your torso curve over completely, releasing your breath. *Repeat 3 times.*

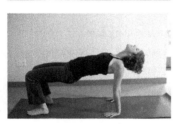

3. **Table.** Lift hips up into table shape on inhale. Keep elbows slightly bent and abdomen in as you open the chest and slowly let the head move back. Come partway down on exhale. Also okay to keep the head forward the whole time. *Repeat 3 times.*

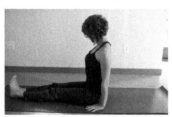

4. **Staff** *(dandasana).* Sit up over sit bones with shoulders above hips. You may need to lift hips up on a blanket and/or bend the knees slightly in order to do this. With heels of the hand at the sides of the hip, reach down through the arms as you lift the sternum. You may need to bend the elbows slightly in order to do this. Simultaneously, reach out through the soles of the feet, so that you are creating two perpendicular vectors reaching out infinitely. Feel the core at work in order to support this dynamic shape. Take 3-5 breaths in this shape.

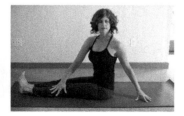

5. **Twisted** *dandasana.* Take one hand over opposite thigh and twist, keeping the spine long and sternum lifted. *Do both sides,* 3-5 breaths.

Repeat sequence 1-5, 3 times.

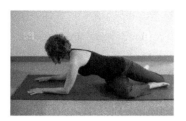

6. **Spiral twist.** Bend one knee in front of you in a half cross-legged position. Bend the other knee back behind you. Sit up tall and twist toward your front leg. Once you have found your natural range of twisting motion, begin to walk the hands forward, keeping the torso long. You may be able to rest on the elbows here. Take 3-5 slow deep breaths against the pressure of the shape. You should feel a deep twist across the abdomen.

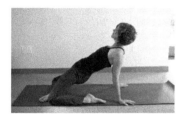

7. **Keeping the legs in the spiral position,** place hands behind hips and lean back into them. Lift hips up on the inhale, reaching the front knee down into the floor to stretch the thigh. Stay for 3-5 breaths. *Repeat on other side.*

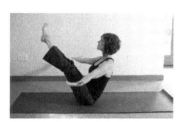

8. **Boat** (*navasana*). Sitting on sit bones, bend knees in front of you. Lift feet off, balancing on sit bones. You can support the legs with the hands behind the knees for a more gentle version, or extend the legs fully to challenge yourself. Keep the chest lifted and shoulders down. Stay for 3-5 breaths. Lower feet and hug knees afterwards, lengthening the spine.

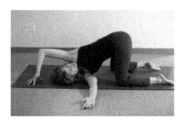

9. **Upper back twist from hands and knees.** Come on to your hands and knees. Place the left palm on the floor directly under the center of the chest and, on the inhale, extend the right hand upwards, twisting the torso to the right. On the exhale, thread the right hand under the left, palm up, and come onto the back of the right shoulder. Looking over the left shoulder relax the right side of the head onto the mat. Take 3-5 deep breaths, relaxing into the earth. *Repeat on other side.*

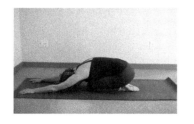

10. **Child's pose** (*balasana*). Reaching the tail bone back, relax forehead to the floor. It is important to relax the belly here, as you have just been twisting and now the blood flow can return and revitalize the digestive area of the body.

Flow sequence *(Vinyasa)*

Vinyasa means "to place in a particular way." In the context of yoga, this means that the poses are smoothly linked together through the breath and consistent awareness. You are noticing and feeling into the movement in between the poses, as much as the poses themselves. This creates an amazing feeling of continuous awareness.

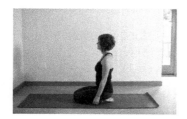

11. Begin this series in kneeling pose (*vajrasana*) - sitting on the shins and knees.

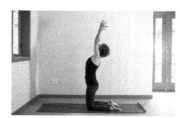

12. Inhale standing up on knees, extending arms up to ears.

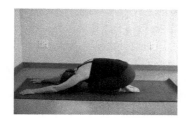

13. Exhale into child's pose.

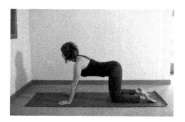

14. Inhale into cow pose. Back is arched, chin is gently lifted.

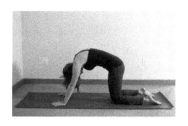

15. Exhale into cat pose. Back is rounded, chin comes down.

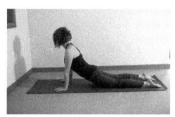

16. Inhale forward into the hands, lowering the pelvis and arching the back gently (gentle upward facing dog with knees on the ground).

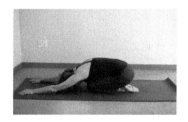

17. Exhale back to child's pose. Take an inhale when you need to, either as you are still moving back into child's pose or resting in the shape.

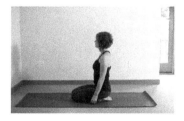

18. Kneeling pose. Exhale, curl the spine up to vertical to finish by sitting on the shins in hero's pose.

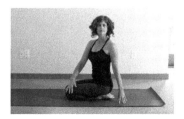

19. Kneeling pose with twist. Sitting on knees and heels, inhale arms up, exhale and twist to one side, bringing arms down. Stay for 3-5 breaths, *then do other side.*

Find a deliberate and graceful pathway up to standing.

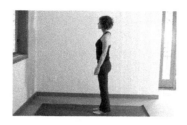

20. Mountain pose (*tadasana*). Stand with feet about hip-width apart, arms relaxed. Feel into your feet - notice the spread of the metatarsal area (at the base of the toes) and the lift of the arches. The abdomen should be engaged, but not extremely so. Chest is open, crown of the head is gently lifted and a feeling of resting the back of the head against an "air pillow" behind you. Move towards ease and a sense of the bones being lined up.

Walk with mindfulness up to the front of your mat. Really feel the feet and toes articulate.

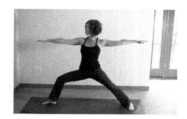

21. Warrior II (*virabhadrasana II*). From mountain pose, bring the hands together in front of the heart. Bend your knees and step the left leg back in line with your left hip, turning the left toes slightly in. Keep the right knee bent directly over the right toes. The left thigh opens outward from the hip and the arms reach out in both directions. The reach from the front and back arm is equal. You want to feel as if you are suspended between your front and back sides.

Transition: Simultaneously straighten your front leg as the right arm extends and right toes turn in. You are now facing sideways on the length of your mat.

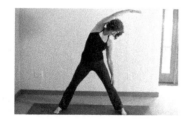

22. Side stretch. Arc the right arm over to your left. Use the core engagement for support.

Transition: Circle right arm in front of face and down to side. Bring heels in, so that both feet are now turned out to approximately 45 degree angles (or to a comfortable angle for your body.)

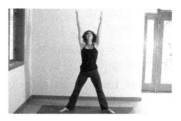

23. **Horse pose with *uddiyana bhanda*.** Inhale arms up to ears, keeping legs extended.

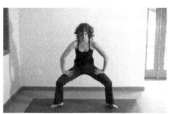

24. **On the exhale,** bend both knees over the toes and bring the arms to thighs. Empty out all of the air and then pull the belly in towards the spine (*uddiyana bandha*), holding the breath out for a second or two. Inhale, straightening the legs and bringing arms up. Exhale and repeat horse with uddiyana bandha after exhale. *Do 3 times.*

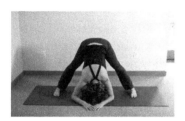

25. **Wide leg forward bend** (*prasarita padotanasana*). Bring toes back to face front. Inhale, press feet into the earth and lift the chest upwards, hands on hips. On the exhale, fold forward at the hips and let the hands come onto the floor (or a block if they don't touch). Stay for 3-5 breaths.

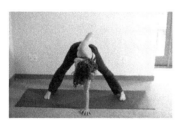

26. **Wide leg forward bend with twist.** Walk hands forward so that they are under the shoulders. Lengthen torso. You may need to come up onto your fingertips or use a block. Bring the left hand under the center of the chest and twist to the right, bringing the right hand up, or to the sacrum. Hold for a couple of breaths, *then do other side.*

Transition: Bend knees, engage the abdomen and round up to standing. Heel-toe the feet back together and mindfully walk back to the front of your mat to stand in mountain pose. Repeat 21-26 on the other side, then gracefully come down to the floor on your belly.

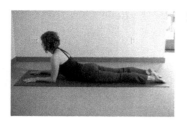

27. **Sphinx**. From the belly, slide forearms forward and rest on elbows and forearms. Take slow deep breaths all the way down into low back. You can also take the elbows out wider if this is causing any strain on your low back. After taking several breaths, let the elbows slide out and then bring arms down to your sides. Turn head to the side.

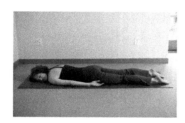

28. **Rest on belly**. This pose is just as important as the last! After squeezing the kidneys and adrenals in the last pose, the release will allow blood to flow back into those areas with volume, nourishing these tissues. Breathe fully into your low back, feeling how the breath can actually stretch the whole low back out.

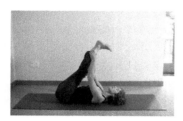

29. **Forward bend on back**. Turn over onto your back and bring the legs up towards the ceiling. You want the ankles to be above the hips. It is okay to bend the knees slightly in order to do this. After a few breaths, reach behind the legs and pull them toward you so that the sit bones lift slightly off the mat. Relax the sit bones down toward the earth. Bend the knees as much as you need to here.

Transition: Hug knees into chest to fully round the back, then stretch out your body on the floor

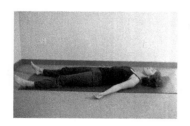

30. **Corpse pose** (*shavasana*). This posture should be comfortable. Get any props you may need to support your body in the shape. You may also want to put on a sweater, socks or blanket to stay warm during this long-held pose. Extend the legs out with feet about one and a half to two feet apart and arms down and a little away from body. You may place a blanket under the head if the chin tends to lift up and/or a rolled blanket under the knees if there is any discomfort in the back. Now, let the whole body drop into the earth, feeling the contact of body and floor. Know you are being held up. No more work to do. Imagine a giant hand of mother earth

holding you completely with benevolence. Let yourself drop into this support. Relax the bones - heavy and earth-like. Relax the connective tissue around the bones. Release the muscles and flesh. Feel even the skin covering the whole body relax. Now relax the mind. This means that while thoughts will come up, you don't need to finish or indulge in them. The mind is simply aware of what is happening, experiencing the body relaxing on earth, moment to moment. Ask yourself every once in a while, "What am I aware of in this moment?"

End the practice by coming up to a short sit, to wake the body up into the calm, alert quality that can feed the rest of your day. This is a wonderful time to do more meditation. Sit as long as you want. Continue to just notice what is happening through all the senses. Do not worry if thoughts come up, such as planning, judging, comparing, wanting, rehearsing, imaginings, etc. Thoughts are just another sensory experience and are unwinding naturally. Just note that they are natural and stay aware of the next experience. You can choose to not indulge in the thought once it has been brought into your awareness. Please see specific meditation guidance in the next section.

Yoga for Cleansing: Full Practice
60-70 minutes

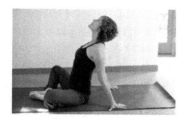

1. **Cobbler (*badha konasana*) with chest opening.** On your inhale, lean back into your hands and open the rib cage, letting the lungs fully open.

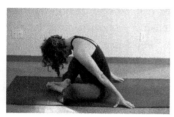

2. **On your exhale,** let your torso curve over completely, releasing your breath. *Repeat 3 times.*

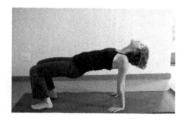

3. **Table.** Lift hips up into table shape on inhale. Keep elbows slightly bent and abdomen in as you open the chest and slowly let the head move back. Come partway down on exhale. Repeat 3 times. Also okay to keep the head forward the whole time.

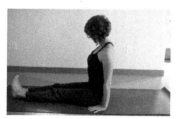

4. **Staff (*dandasana*).** Sit up over sit bones with shoulders above hips. You may need to lift hips up on a blanket and/ or bend the knees slightly in order to do this. With heels of the hands at the sides of the hip, reach down through the arms as you lift the sternum bone. You may need to bend the elbows slightly in order to do this. Simultaneously, reach out through the soles of the feet, so that you are creating two perpendicular vectors reaching out infinitely. Feel the core at work in order to support this dynamic shape. Take 3-5 breaths.

Repeat numbers 1-4, 2 times

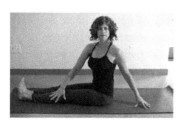

5. **Twisted** *dandasana*. Take one hand over opposite thigh and twist, keeping the spine long and sternum lifted. *Do both sides*, 3-5 breaths.

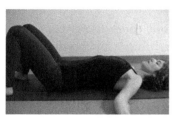

6. **Pelvic tilts on back**. Move onto back. Massage area under rib cage and make circles around belly. Keep hands on belly and feel the breath move into hands. After several breaths, on the exhale engage the belly and move it in towards the spine as if you were trying to zip up tight jeans. The low back will flatten towards the floor. On inhale, relax belly and let the spine return to its natural curve. *Do about 5 of these slowly.*

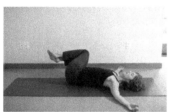

7. **Wringing out the spine**. Bring knees in towards you with arms straight out to the sides of body. Twist partway to one side, then exhale, pull belly in and bring knees back to vertical. On inhale, move to other side. Keep moving slowly back and forth, increasing the range of motion as ready. Feel your weight moving across the back of the pelvis, massaging that part of the body. Stay interested in the experience of the body.

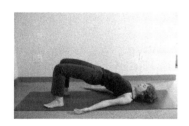

8. **Shoulder bridge**. Bringing feet to floor, hip width apart, lift hips up. The arms can come down to your sides, palms up. Feel your feet spread and the action of the legs moving toward each other. Take slow steady breaths.

Transition: Lower butt, till it is relaxed, then reach sit bones towards heels as you lower, lengthening the spine. Interlace hands behind head and curl up into a low sit up. Let the head rest into the palms of hands. Slip the thumbs under the occiput, the bony protuberances at the base of both sides of head. Gently push in with thumbs and extend head away from hips as you lower down, lengthening the upper spine.

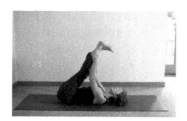

9. **Forward bend on back.** Turn over onto your back and bring the legs up toward the ceiling. You want the ankles to be above the hips. It is okay to bend the knees slightly in order to do this. After a few breaths, reach behind the legs and pull them toward you so that the sit bones lift slightly off the mat. Relax the sit bones down toward the earth. Bend the knees as much as you need to here.

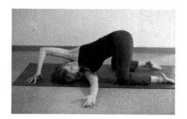

10. **Upper back twist from hands and knees.** Come on to your hands and knees. On the inhale, bring left hand under the center of the chest and extend the right hand upwards, twisting the torso to the right. On the exhale, thread right hand under the left, palm up, and come onto the back of the right shoulder. Looking over the left shoulder, relax the right side of the head onto the mat. Take 3-5 deep breaths relaxing into the earth. *Repeat on other side.*

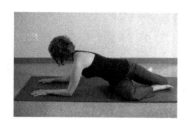

11. **Spiral twist.** Bend one knee in front of you in a half cross-legged position. Then bend the other knee back behind you. Sit up tall and twist toward your front leg. Once you have found your natural range of twisting motion, begin to walk the hands forward, keeping the torso long. You may be able to rest on the elbows here. Take 3-5 slow deep breaths against the pressure of the shape. You should feel a deep twist across the abdomen.

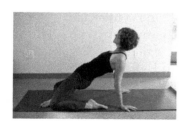

12. **Keeping the legs in the spiral position**, place hands behind hips and lean back into them. Lift hips up on the inhale, reaching the front knee down into the floor to stretch the thigh. *Do the other side.*

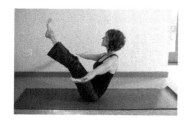

13. **Boat Pose** (*navasana*). Sitting on sit bones, bend knees in front of you. Lift feet off, balancing on sit bones. You can support the legs with the hands behind the knees for a gentler version or extend the legs fully to challenge yourself. Keep the chest lifted and shoulders down. Take 3-5 breaths. Lower feet and hug knees afterwards, lengthening the spine.

Transition: Swing legs around, stretch feet and roll up to standing.

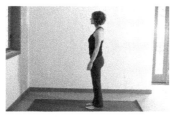

14. Mountain pose (*tadasana*). Stand with feet about hip-width apart, arms relaxed. Feel into your feet - notice the spread of the metatarsal area (at the base of the toes) and the lift of the arches. The abdomen should be engaged, but not extremely so. Chest is open, crown of the head is gently lifted and feel a resting of the back of the head against an "air pillow" behind you. Move toward ease and a sense of the bones being lined up. Walk with mindfulness up to the front of your mat. Really feel the feet and toes articulate.

Simple *Vinyasa*

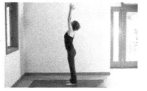

15. Inhale, arms extending up to ears.

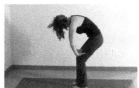

16. Exhale, bend knees and bring hands to thighs, rounding back

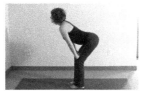

17. Inhale, arch back.

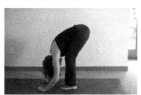

18. Exhale, release upper body over the legs.

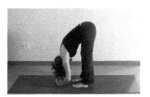

19. Inhale and extend sit bones to the ceiling while reaching the heels to the earth.

Transition: Exhale, soften knees and round up, engaging the abdomen and keeping neck and shoulders soft. Feel your feet the whole way up. Repeat vinyasa sequence 3 times.

Sun salutation (*Surya namaskar*)

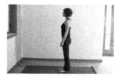

20. Start in mountain pose.

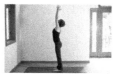

21. Inhale arms up, reach up to ears.

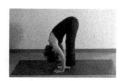

22. Exhale, bend forward over legs.

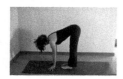

23. Half forward bend (*ardha uttinasana*). Inhale, extend torso forward from the sides of body. Keep neck long.

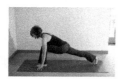

24. Exhale, step right leg back to lunge. Stay in the shape on the inhale, extending from the back heel to the crown of the head.

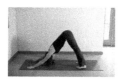

25. Exhale, step back into *adho mukha shwanasana* (downward facing dog).

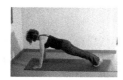

26. Inhale to plank.

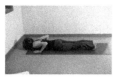

27. Exhale, bend elbows and lower body down to the floor in one piece. (You can bend knees to floor if you want.)

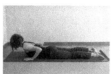

28. Inhale to cobra pose. Bend elbows so hands are under shoulders and lift chest. Keep neck long.

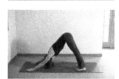

29. Exhale, push yourself back into downward dog. You can push up to plank first or move back through bent knees.

Inhale, stay in the down dog shape.

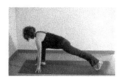

30. Exhale, step your right foot forward between hands. (On second round, you will step first with the left foot.)

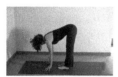

31. Step the left foot forward all the way to front of mat, extending torso back into *ardha uttinasana*.

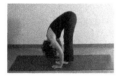

32. Exhale to forward bend.

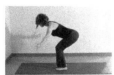

33. Bend the knees slightly, lift the chest and inhale up to standing with the abdomen engaged and the arms reaching up to the ears.

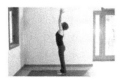

Let your hands rest together at heart for one breath. Repeat the sequence, stepping the left foot when moving into and out of the lunges.

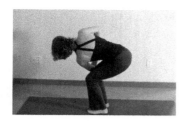

34. Revolved chair (*parivrtta utkatnasana*). Inhale arms up to ears. On the exhale, bring hands together in front of the heart while bending knees. Lean forward a little and engage the abdomen. Bring the left elbow over the right thigh and gently push the right hand down on the left, twisting to your right. On each inhale, lengthen the sides of the waist. On each exhale, bring the abdomen muscles into the body. Hold for 3-5 breaths, *then do other side.*

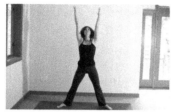

35. Horse pose with *uddiyana bhanda*. Inhale arms up to ears, keeping legs extended.

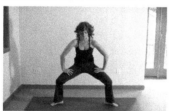

36. On the exhale, bend both knees over the toes and bring the arms to thighs. Empty out all of the air and then pull the belly in towards the spine (*uddiyana bandha*), holding the breath out for a second or two. Inhale, straightening the legs and bringing arms up. Exhale and repeat horse with uddiyana bandha after exhale. *Do 3 times.*

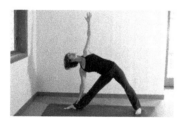

37. Extended Triangle. From horse pose, turn in your left foot and turn the right foot so that it is parallel to the length of your mat. Straighten both legs and extend arms out to the sides, grounding into both feet. Extend the right arm forward, lengthening under the right rib cage. Keeping torso over the legs, place right hand down on right leg. Extend left arm upwards focusing on the left hand or straight side. Relax shoulders down and open chest and upper back wide. Drop back into the back body, bringing right inner thigh forward and left thigh back. Push energetically into both feet while reaching up through upper arm to come up. *Repeat horse pose, and then do the other side for extended triangle.*

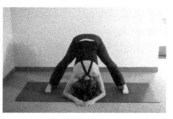

38. Wide-leg forward bend (*prasarita padotanasana*). Bring toes to face front. Inhale, press feet into the earth and lift the chest upwards, hands on hips. On the exhale, fold forward at the hips and let the hands come onto the floor, or a block if they don't touch. Stay for 3-5 breaths.

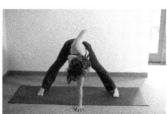

39. Wide-leg forward bend with twist. Walk hands forward so that they are under the shoulders. Lengthen torso. You may need to come up onto your fingertips or use a block. Bring the left hand under the center of the chest and twist to the right, bringing the right hand up, or to the sacrum. Hold for a couple of breaths, *then do other side.*

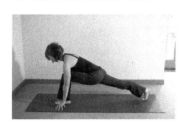

40. Twisted lunge. Walk hands over toward right foot while turning right foot parallel to length of mat, with one hand on each side of the right foot. The back heel is up. Keep left hand on the mat. Engage abdomen up into body and twist to the right, keeping the pelvis stable. Extend right arm up or keep at sacrum. *(*Note: second side is pictured here.)*

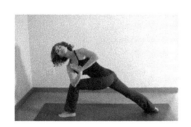

41. Twisted lunge - Going deeper. Place right hand on right thigh. Bring left elbow across right thigh, placing right hand on top of left in front of heart. Try to bring left heel down to floor with foot at an angle. Breathe long into the spine and use core strength. *Return to lunge and bring hands to the inside of the front leg. Turn front foot in and return to wide-leg forward bend. Repeat 38 and 39, and then go into twisted lunge on the second side. (*Note: second side is pictured here.)*

Transition: To come up, bend knees, ground into feet, engage abdomen and place hands on thighs. Lift chest and come up to vertical. Heel-toe feet back together and stand at the front of your mat.

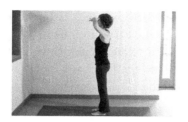

42. Pranic scan. Inhale arms up to ears. On the exhale, bend elbows with fingers pointing in towards each other and scan down the front of body. Keep your hands very close to, but not touching, the body, so you can feel heat and energy emanating from your body. Hands stop when your exhale ends. Take another inhale and on the exhale resume the body scan. The idea is to feel the energy smoothly move down the body. Once the hands are extended down at your sides, continue to visualize energy moving down the legs into the soles of the feet. Feel the earth under you.

Transition: Make your way gracefully onto your belly.

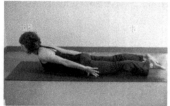

43. Locust pose (*shalabasana*). With arms down at your sides, lift the chest head and legs. Keep the back of hands lightly resting on the floor. Keep your neck long and think about lengthening out through the legs and crown of head. Stay for 3-5 breaths. Relax down for a couple of breaths, turning your head to one side. *(Locust with extended arms shown here.)*

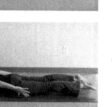

44. Locust pose with extended arms. Take *shalabasana* one more time. This time, when you lift the chest and legs, also extend the arms towards your feet, palms facing into body. Relax down onto your belly for a couple breaths, turning your head to the other side.

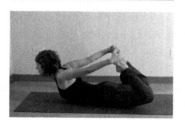

45. Bow pose (*dhanurasana*). Bend your knees and grab a hold of your feet. Open the front of your hip bones toward the floor. On an inhale, lift the chest and thighs, kicking feet into the palms of your hands. Easy gaze at the end of nose. Stay for 3-5 breaths.   Rest on your belly for a couple of breaths, deeply breathing into the back body.

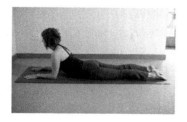

46. Sphinx. From the belly, slide forearms forward and rest on elbows and forearms. Take slow deep breaths all the way down into low back. You can also take the elbows out wider if this is causing any strain on your low back. Hold for 5 breaths.

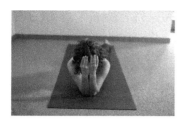

47. Sphinx with head hold. Walk elbows together so that they are touching, or as close together as possible. Walk elbows forward or slide body back till you feel a slight stretch through the shoulders and arms. Turn palms up. Lift head up and place thumbs on the inner eyebrows, so that your whole head is resting into your thumbs. Stay for several breaths. This will apply some pressure to the *marma* points located here. Marma points are energetic places in the body that link body and consciousness. This marma point can help prevent and mitigate headaches.

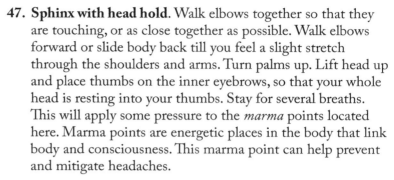

48. Sphinx with head hold (part 2). Bring chin down and slowly slide thumbs along eyebrows laterally. When the thumbs reach the temples, drop the top of head into palms and completely hold your head. Let worries and struggles spill out of the head into your palms.

Transition: Lift head, move elbows apart and come down onto belly. Bring hands under shoulders, gently lift yourself up and push back so that you are on your hands and knees. Bring your big toes together and knees wide then walk hands in so that you are sitting on your heels.

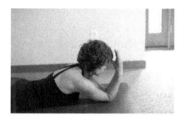

49. Marma pressure at small intestine (easy *mayurasana*). As you exhale, turn knuckles in toward your center. Inhale and reach arms straight out in front of you. Turn palms up and make fists with your hands. Bend elbows and bring fists right inside the front of your hip bones.

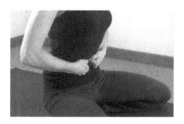

50. Marma pressure with forward bend. Turn knuckles in toward your center as you fold over hands in child's pose. Your forehead can rest on the floor. Breathe up against the pressure at your small intestine caused by the hands. Stay for several breaths. Curl up and release hands.

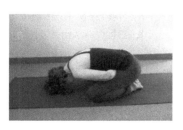

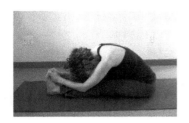

51. **Seated forward bend** (*paschimotanasana*). Bring legs around to the front of you and rock from side to side, moving the flesh out from under the buttocks. Sit up tall, lengthening the front body. Walk hands forward at sides of legs and fold forward from the hips. After several breaths, and as long as your weight is forward of the sit bones, release the back and head and either take a hold of feet or keep hands at your sides. On each inhale, think of extending the sit bones back behind you while lengthening the whole spine. On the exhale, relax forward over legs. Keep the abdomen soft. Stay for 9 breaths.

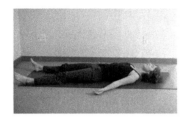

52. **Corpse pose** (*shavasana*). This posture should be comfortable. Get any props you may need to support your body in the shape. You may also want to put on a sweater, socks or blanket to stay warm during this long-held pose. Extend the legs out with feet about 1 ½ - 2 feet apart and arms down and a little away from body. You may place a blanket under the head if the chin tends to lift up and/or a rolled blanket under the knees if there is any discomfort in the back. Now, let the whole body drop into the earth, feeling the contact of body and floor. Know you are being held up. No more work to do. Imagine a giant hand of mother earth holding you completely with benevolence. Let yourself drop into this support. Relax the bones - heavy and earth-like. Relax the connective tissue around the bones. Release the muscles and flesh. Feel even the skin covering the whole body relax. Now relax the mind. This means that while thoughts will come up, you don't need to finish or indulge in them. The mind is simply aware of what is happening, experiencing the body relaxing on earth, moment to moment. Ask yourself every once in a while, "What am I aware of in this moment?

End the practice by coming up to a short seat. Just check-in again. Notice the balance of effort and ease - that calm yet alert quality. Keep tasting the effect of your practice and make an intention to carry any ease, clarity, awareness and sattva into your day.

MEDITATION FOR CLEANSING

Meditation is a practice for cultivating healthy states of mind. We practice focusing the mind so that it is disciplined enough to steadily observe what is happening in our lives with a longer attention span. And, we practice mindfulness - noticing what is happening as it is happening - so that we can be fully present to our lives. While there are many types of meditation, here we share a couple of simple practices you can do daily during this cleanse and beyond.

The practice itself nurtures our capacity to focus and be mindful, so that the more we practice, the easier it is to practice and the more natural it feels to be present and aware. Once we have a mind that is gathered, we have the capability of being with things as they are happening. For example, instead of replaying a conversation from the past while taking a walk outside, we have the opportunity to be mindful and experience the sensory gifts of the natural world. Mindfulness interrupts that haze of mind chatter. In that pause of awareness, we are not adding to the unconscious thoughts. This is freedom. In this moment of clarity, we are no longer a naïve victim of our thoughts and old stories. We start to notice the connection between our thoughts and emotions and how they play out in the body. In the pause of awareness, we can make real-time choices about our actions.

We hope you can already see the tremendous benefits mindfulness can have on our eating and health choices. The truth is, most of us have a good idea what it takes to be healthy, but are often governed by unhealthy habits born from unconscious thinking.

There are many ways and avenues into meditation. If you already have a sitting practice, carry on. Having this practice in place during the cleanse will help you stay steady through any emotions and physical changes that come about during the cleanse. It will offer you a calm respite from the busyness of your day. It may offer insight, wisdom and compassion in dealing with your personality, stories and habits. These guided practices below are meant to get you started, and then you can stay with the meditation as long as you like. We recommend starting with something manageable, perhaps 5-10 minutes. You can then build up to 20-40 minutes. Consistency is important, so finding guilt-free time and space is key.

Practice 1: Focusing on the Breath

First, make yourself comfortable in a sitting posture. We really mean that. So, sit against a wall if you need to, add cushions under your seat, sit in a chair. Do whatever you can do to allow the spine to be erect and dignified, but without being in pain. If necessary, it is also okay to do this one lying down. Give yourself permission to fully be here. Know that all those things on the "to do" list can wait. Let yourself explore the practice of awareness.

Drop your awareness into your body and notice the shape of it: the feeling of weight in your hips, how you have placed your arms and legs, the angle of your wrists and fingers, the space around the body. Now notice the temperature of the body, where it is warm, where it is cool. Notice places that feel snug and taut and the places that feel loose and relaxed in the body. Imagine you have just put on this body suit and are noticing how it fits. Is it tight in the shoulders? Just right in the waist? Without needing to fix it, really notice and feel being in this body. Accept it all as it is.

Now notice the breath in the body – just noticing it, not needing to change it. Pay particular attention to the geography of the breath: where and how you feel it in the body as you are breathing, the sense of the ribs moving, the belly, the chest. Feel the air across the nostrils. Hone in on one of these physical aspects where you feel the breath most vividly. Stay with these sensations for several breaths.

Now begin noticing the temporal quality of the breath. Notice how long the inhale seems to be taking, and the exhale. Are there pauses? Feel the four parts of the breath and how they move through time and space: the inhale, the tiny pause/transition to exhale, the exhale and the tiny moment of emptiness at the bottom of the exhale. You are still feeling the physical geography of the breath, but are now adding this temporal quality to it. Stay with several breaths, feeling the sensations of breath in the body and the rhythm of each breath.

Now begin noticing the quality of each breath. Each breath is like a brush stroke of paint: sometimes it feels smooth, sometimes jagged, or anything in between. Each moment of the breath is different. Is it thin or wide, a whisper or broad like a full wave? Stay with several breaths, noticing their quality.

Now feel all three of these aspects. Breath by breath, feel the movement in the body, how it is moving temporally and the quality of each breath along its wave. Breath by breath. Experience it fully. Each breath. Riding it fully to the top of the inhale and all the way to the bottom of the exhale.

Now, step into the center of the breath, so that the breath is breathing you now. You are completely inside the breath. Relax into this for several minutes.

When you are ready, come back to feeling the shape of your body. Then notice the space around the body, the sense of the room, sounds, temperature, smells. Slowly open your eyes and just feel. Give yourself a moment to "taste" the effect of your practice. This quality and awareness that you have right now is part of your nature. Know you can access it whenever you remember. And practice helps you remember.

Practice 2: Open Awareness Meditation
This is simply the practice of becoming familiar with the quality of awareness. We will start with some simple concentration practices, pointing back out to the feeling of awareness with each one. We will then allow the object of focus to be unselected - a flow of information coming through the senses and the mind. We love this practice because it is very transferable to everyday life. You can move from this type of meditation into your life seamlessly.

As always, take a moment to make yourself comfortable, sitting on a cushion, sitting in a chair, or even lying, so that the body is comfortable, but alert! Land in this body. Bring all your attention into this body. Almost as if you came from another planet and you are inhabiting and feeling this body for the first time. What is it like to be in this body today? Feeling immediate simple sensations like warmth, coolness, movement, static, tingling, density, numbness, energy, hunger, sleepiness, ease, etc. Not needing to change it – just noticing.

In this moment, as you are noticing this, you are aware of your body. Feel the feeling of awareness. Aware of the body. You are here with it.

And now let your attention move to the breath in the body. Notice where you feel the breath opening the body and then releasing it through the exhale. Feel the shape and timing of each breath. Really become interested in the breath. How is it moving through your body from the beginning to the end? From that first moment the breath enters the body, to the top of the inhale, to the full exhale all the way to the bottom, feel into that moment before you begin a new breath. Stay with several breaths. In this moment, you are aware of breathing. Feel that quality of awareness. Notice being here, with your breath.

Now bring your attention to the center of the chest and your heart. Notice that physical part of the body. Notice if there are any moods, feelings. They might be very subtle or more overt. You don't have to figure out what it is or conjure up a feeling. There is always something, even if its just neutral or boredom. Take a few minutes to notice feelings and mood.
In this moment you are aware of the feeling tones in the body. Feel into this awareness. You are with your feelings.

Now bring your attention to the mind and thoughts. Just waiting and paying attention so that you may notice a thought arising, or even the subtle feeling of wanting to think a thought. Sometimes you will notice the thought after you've been involved in it for a while. Maybe you have been caught up in a story. That's okay. When you notice, in that moment, you are aware of the mind. Let yourself stay with this observing of thoughts for a while. Also, notice the space and time between thoughts when the mind feels still and quiet.

In this moment you are aware of the mind. Feel that awareness. Let yourself get familiar with this noticing quality.

And now, let yourself relax into this quality of noticing...without an agenda. Now you can open up the lens and let whatever comes into your awareness be known. You don't have to go out and find something or direct your awareness. Just sit back and relax. See what comes to you. Sometimes it's a sound or a body sensation, a thought or feeling. They are all just flowing through you. A stream of morphing phenomena. Nothing to push away. Nothing to create. Everything is fair game. Even this. Relaxing. Staying interested. Feel the stream of life move through you.

Feel your body again. Notice having a body, then slowly let your eyes open, letting the awareness of vision come in – light, shapes, colors. Notice the whole world freshly appearing in each moment again and again. Each moment is a new, fresh experience.

Now you can simply move from this practice right into your day, letting this awareness carry into your doing and not-doing. Remember to notice as much as possible. You might start to notice things you normally take for granted, like the feel of your hands on the steering wheel as you drive, or the feeling of the hot water on your body as you shower. Choose something you do on a daily basis and practice this mindfulness with it. Doing this consistently creates a portal to awareness. Its like re-wiring the brain so that when you do that task, instead of getting lost in unconscious thinking, you suddenly remember to notice and be with the moment. Every once in a while, you might need to close your eyes and come back into the body to narrow down the focus because there are so many things to be aware of in the fullness of our lives. As we get more and more familiar with awareness, wisdom takes over and we know what to focus on, what to be aware of. We learn this.

PRANAYAMA FOR CLEANSING

The pranayama practice for cleansing is made up of three breathing practices: *Kapal bhati*, *Agni sara dhati* and *Ashwini mudra*. We recommend doing the breathing exercises daily during all phases of the Mindbody Cleanse. You can view videos of these three practices at meadowheartayurveda.com. These three practices clear and balance all three doshas in this order: kapha – upper respiratory tract; pitta – small intestine; and vata – colon. These practices are extremely beneficial for digestion and elimination during cleansing. These pranayama techniques should be practiced within your comfort zone and without strain.

You will do three rounds of each type of breathing practice. Take one full breath in between rounds. Once you finish three rounds, you can sit quietly feeling the breath. Notice the effect in your physiology and state of mind. Take your time in between each practice, taking several slow, easy breaths before moving to the next practice.

Before beginning the three practices below, sit in an upright, comfortable position. Take some time to tune into your breath with relaxed awareness before you begin.

1) *Kapal bhati* (skull shining): In this practice you take several (10 - 50) short, quick exhalations through the nose while bringing in the belly sharply. A passive inhale happens through the nose between each exhale. To start, take a breath in and then release half of the air out. Bring the belly in, in a sharp, quick manner to complete the exhale. Let the inhale happen naturally, allowing the belly to relax. Continue to bring the belly in with a short quick motion on the exhale and release the belly with a passive inhale. This creates a "bounce" feeling through the belly and you will hear each exhale. Find a consistent rhythm that feels comfortable to you. Usually it will be slightly faster than

one breath per second. You will take at least 10 breaths like this and can build up to 50+. You will do three rounds of these 10 - 50 breaths, taking a slow, full breath in between each round.

2) *Agnisara dhauti* (cleansing the digestive fire): Start by sitting on your heels with the knees wide or in supported *virasana*. You can also do this practice standing, with the feet wider than your hips and the knees bent. Inhale fully through the nose. As you exhale through the nose, lean forward onto your hands and knees (or place your hands on your thighs if you are standing) and empty the lungs completely. Holding your breath ***out***, bring the belly in deeply toward the spine. Next, relax the belly all the way out. Bring the belly in deeply again with strength and then release all the way again. Think of "pumping" the belly in strongly, then releasing, then pumping in and releasing again. Do this as many times as possible with comfort, without taking in a new breath. Usually about three to ten times is comfortable for most people. It is important to not strain

while holding the breath out and without gasping for air when you inhale. As you inhale, sit upright again and take one comfortable breath. Repeat another two rounds until you have done a total of three rounds.

3) *Ashwini mudra* (horse seal): Inhale deeply and hold your breath *in*. Bring your chin down to your chest (*jalandhara bhanda*). With the breath still held in, squeeze in and pull up on the anal sphincter muscle around the anus, then relax it. Repeat this three to ten times, or as many times as is comfortable, without exhaling, at approximately the same pace as the belly "pumping" from *agnisara dhauti*. When you feel ready, bring your head up to vertical and exhale. Take one full breath and then repeat until you have completed three rounds.

When you have finished all three practices, three times each, sit quietly letting the breath be natural and unguided. Taste the effect on your body, energy and mind state.

Chapter 6
Self Care

"The idea is not to perfect yourself – you've already tried that – the idea is to perfect your love, your kindness."

– Jack Kornfield

We can't emphasize enough how important it is to schedule relaxation time throughout the cleanse. Remember, traditional PK is residential, where there is ample time for relaxation. It is when we feel safe, relaxed and nurtured that the stubborn emotional layers will release. We want to create that same container in our home cleanse, to the best of our ability. We recommend actually scheduling time in your day for relaxation. Some ideas are:

- Longer, more relaxed meal times
- Time away from technology/work
- Walking in nature
- Journaling, drawing
- Extra sleep
- Sitting and enjoying a cup of digestive tea

Aside from this relaxation time, there are several other self-care practices that support a complete Mindbody Cleanse.

ESSENTIAL SELF-CARE PRACTICES

Self-massage with oil (abhyanga)

During this cleanse we recommend practicing daily self-massage with oil. You probably already use some type of lotion or moisturizer after you bathe. However, when you replace this habit with high quality oil, you not only keep the skin supple and moist, but also coat the nerves that lie just below the skin's surface. Nerve cells need good fat to stay healthy and this ritual will help stabilize and calm the nervous system. In addition, you avoid the many added chemicals, stabilizers and fragrances in most lotions that block the channels of the body. Purchase high quality

organic oil that you prefer such as sesame, almond, sunflower or coconut. Traditionally, abhyanga is done with warm herbal oil which you can get from Ayurvedic supply sites (see page 98). Oil allows the herbs to penetrate more deeply into the tissues and you can find oils specifically suited to PK and detoxification.

Before your shower or bath, coat the whole body with the oil, using long strokes over muscles and circular motions around joints. Apply in the direction of hair growth. When looking down at your body, make clockwise circles around your belly and chest. After applying oil, it is best to wait 10 - 15 minutes before getting into the bath or shower. In the first five minutes, the skin absorbs the oil and for every minute after that, the next tissue layer will be saturated. Because there are seven tissue layers, this time frame allows all layers of tissue to benefit from the oiling process. If you don't have time, don't worry - you will still benefit from the oil. You can add a light coat of oil after your bath or shower, before you dress, as well. Self massage is a great way to nurture self-love.

Oils for Self Massage

It is best to use an Ayurvedic herbal oil blend. In lieu of that, an all-natural, cold-pressed, organic oil can be used for self massage. Everything you put on your skin ends up in your bloodstream, so it is important to only use oils that are safe for ingestion. The best oil for you may depend on your constitutional type, however, during cleansing sesame oil is good for all types. Another idea is to add essential oils to a base oil. While these do not offer the benefits that herbs do, their scents

Massage Oils and Essential Oils by Constitution Type

Vata

Use a base of sesame, avocado or castor oil (or any combination of these).
Grounding, warming and sweet scents balance vata.

Good essential oils for vata include:

- Clove
- Orange
- Lavender
- Vetiver
- Frankincense
- Bergamot
- Cinnamon
- Neroli
- Patchouli
- Sweet orange
- Ylang ylang
- Vanilla

Pitta

Use a base of sunflower, coconut or sesame oil (or a combination of any of these).
Cooling, calming and sweet scents balance pitta.

Good essential oils for pitta include:

- Rose
- Jasmine
- Rose geranium
- Fennel
- Sandalwood
- Peppermint
- Chamomile
- Clary Sage
- Lemon balm
- Lemongrass
- Lime
- Neroli
- Vanilla

Kapha

Use a base of sunflower, mustard or almond oil (or a combination of any of these).
Warming and stimulating scents benefit kapha.

Good essential oils for kapha include:

- Camphor
- Eucalyptus
- Myrrh
- Holy Basil (Tulsi)
- Rosemary
- Sage
- Bergamot
- Fir
- Grapefruit
- Juniper
- Neroli
- Sweet Orange

can make the oiling process even more enjoyable. The previous page offers suggested base oils and essential oils you can add to your base oil specific to dosha type. Of course, the nose knows! If you are drawn to a particular scent that isn't on your "list," trust your instinct before you trust a list!

Daily Baths

We recommend daily Epsom salt baths during the Purification Phase of your cleanse. You will do the self-abhyanga massage followed by a warm bath with Epsom salts. This is our at-home *svedana* (therapeutic sweating) practice. In addition, the Epsom salts help draw toxins from the body. The bath also gives you some scheduled quiet relaxation time. Many folks mention that this is their favorite cleanse ritual.

No bathtub? No worries. You can do the self-abhyanga massage before your hot shower and practice the meditation of showering, noticing the whole ritual of a shower: the feel of the water, the smell and texture of soap, the air on your wet skin, your towel and clothing.

Exercise

A little bodily movement each day is beneficial during your cleanse. Exercise helps balance blood sugar levels and moves the lymph. It stimulates sweating, which is another form of natural detoxification. Exercise also improves metabolism and agni, the digestive fire. If you normally have a very rigorous work-out routine, you may want to ease back a little. Cleansing is a time of releasing, not building, so you may notice you feel more tired or your muscles feel weak. Listen to your body and accept your

limits. If you are someone who does not already have a daily movement routine, please make sure to take a walk and/or practice some yoga each day.

OPTIONAL SELF-CARE PRACTICES

The following are practices that greatly increase the benefits of your home cleanse. Integrate these as much as possible.

Steam Sauna

In traditional panchakarma, you would receive steam treatments following a professional abhyanga massage. This is referred to as *svedana*, therapeutic sweating. So, if you have access to a steam sauna during your home cleanse, you can do the self-abhyanga prior to taking your sauna.

Professional Abhyanga Massage

Getting back to our benchmark of trying to emulate PK as much as possible, it is highly recommended to receive a professional abhyanga massage during the cleanse if possible. If you are only able to get one professional abhyanga massage, the best time for scheduling it will be days four to seven of the Purification Phase. Traditionally, this massage is done with two therapists working in tandem. In addition to using copious amounts of warm herbal oil all over the body, *marma* points are stimulated through gentle touch. *Marma* points are very similar to acupuncture points but are accessed with touch instead of needles. These points on the body are where consciousness and matter meet, encouraging the release of deeply held emotions and openings in the channels of the body. According to Dr. Vasant Lad in *Textbook of Ayurveda*, "In panchakarma, application of oil to the skin goes into the deeper tissues, *mamsa dhatu*, and begins releasing repressed emotions...The subtle quality of sesame oil helps to release emotions by stimulating certain neurotransmitters in the central nervous system. Because of oil massage, those crystals of unresolved emotions become decrystalized and dissolve."

Shirodhara

Shirodhara is typically part of a PK protocol, as it is a profound treatment for relaxation, restoration of the nerves, and release of deeply stored emotions. *Shiro* means head and *dhara* means flow. A mix of warmed sesame oil and herbs specific to the nervous system is poured in a steady stream onto the forehead for approximately 30 minutes. Shirodhara improves circulation to the brain, reduces stress and anxiety and is especially helpful in nervous system imbalances such as insomnia, anxiety, chronic fatigue, and IBS. We highly recommend you schedule this treatment in conjunction with your Ayurvedic home cleanse.

Counseling

The cleanse is conducive to self-reflection. It may be useful for you to see your counselor during or after the process of cleansing to maximize this time of increased self-awareness.

Other Bodywork Therapies

Bodywork is wonderful to have during the whole cleanse process. Keep in mind that you want gentle therapies that encourage the opening of channels in the body for the release of stored emotions and toxins. The Ayurvedic therapies, such as abhyanga and shirodhara are especially designed to encourage this opening and subsequent release, and are the best compliment to your home cleanse. However, other therapies, especially if they are already part of your self-care routine, may be useful to schedule during the cleanse as well. These therapies may include: acupuncture, gentle massage (you can always bring your own oil along for the massage therapist to use, if you do not have access to an Ayurvedic practitioner), craniosacral massage and energy work, such as reiki, Emotional Freedom Technique or Healing Touch.

WORKING WITH EMOTIONS

Emotions come up during the cleanse as they are being mobilized out of the body. It is important to digest and fully release them. In Ayurveda tears are understood to be another form of self-cleansing. We want to encourage you to let emotions flow through you during your cleanse. This reiterates the necessity for clearing plenty of space in your schedule during this mind and body cleanse.

Often we get stuck in patterns with emotions. And when we haven't learned to work with them, these emotional waves have a way of taking us under. To change this pattern, we must have enough awareness to break out of the story and thoughts that are reinforcing the emotional turmoil. In a moment of awareness, we can see and feel what is happening without adding to its magnitude. We can learn to find a calm presence behind the emotion and then ride the emotional wave. Ultimately, if you stay aware as much as possible through the emotions, you will begin to draw from this experience. You will develop a confidence in your ability to handle difficult emotions. As you accumulate experiences in riding these waves of emotion, you teach yourself a new way of responding to them. This wisdom will enter into your response when they arise the next time around as you develop your own way of working with them. The following are suggestions in working with emotions that have come out of our studies in Yoga and Buddhism.

There are 4 basic parts to this awareness approach. Once you are familiar with these tools, they may even become a mantra that you can say to yourself as a reminder when emotions come up. Over time this will feel less contrived and you will improvise these steps and their order, finding your own pathway.

The 4 tools are: Acknowledge, Feel, Calm, Understand.

1) *Acknowledge the emotion.* Don't judge the emotion as wrong, bad or excessive. It is natural. Remind yourself that the emotion is universal. All emotions, difficult and positive, are a part of the human experience and are experienced in similar ways. So, instead of referring to the emotion as "my grief" or "I am angry," you can say something like, "grief is moving through me" or "anger is here." It really isn't ours. It is a common emotional experience that moves through our form in a given span of time. This allows us to feel more connected

and compassionate toward others when they, too, are going through that emotion. When we identify with it as ours, this misleads us into thinking it is a permanent part of our being.

2) *Feel the emotion in your body.* Yes, actually let yourself feel how the emotion is affecting your physical form. Is there tightness and constriction in the body? Where do you feel it? How does the breath feel? Is there a ball of nerves in the gut or throat? There is no "right" answer here – the sensation may be in your arms or hands – just notice where in your physical body you can feel the emotion. Stay with it as long as you can, just feeling it without going back to the story and circumstances. If this is too overwhelming, move on to Part 3.

3) *Find calm by moving your attention to a neutral object.* Focus your awareness on something that does not trigger an emotional response. This could be the breath, feeling a neutral or relaxed sensation in the body, focusing on sounds, or going outside and taking in nature through the senses.

Another helpful approach is to try vigorous physical movement. The stress hormones were created for this purpose, such as running from a threatening situation, so physical movement will help dissipate the stress-fighting chemicals in the body. Go for a brisk walk or hike. Alternatively, you can do a yoga practice. In your practice, start with flowing standing poses, like sun salutations, keeping an even, full breath in the forefront of your practice. Once you feel more settled, try holding the poses longer and do an inversion like *viparita karani* (legs up the wall, perpendicular to torso), a shoulder stand or a shoulder bridge on a block.

4) *Understand what happened.* When the mind is calm, revisit the experience. What was the specific memory or story that led to the emotion? What triggered the emotion? Watch this memory play in your mind from your neutral standpoint. Notice the feeling of calm now that you are no longer in that difficult moment. Acknowledge that you are here, while the event that triggered the strong emotional response happened in another time and place that is not happening now.

Notice if you get caught up in the story and drama of it. If so, move back through the proceeding steps again. As you investigate the experience, you will see that the emotion was a natural response based on all the previous causes and conditions in your life thus far. You will be able to hold compassion for yourself by understanding the difficulties of the experience. Don't worry about getting this right. You may not be able to get to calm and understand right away. This is okay. Just keep noticing – you will eventually begin to see more and more, thus developing more skill in handling emotions. On the other hand, with practice, you may notice yourself being able to move through this process more and more quickly. You may even be able to acknowledge the emotion and then immediately move to understanding.

A note about positive emotions
This often gets left in the dust, but during the cleanse, you may also experience some very pleasant emotions. Again, acknowledge and feel into the physical experience of the emotion. In this way, it becomes a vivid experience for you to draw from. Feel any gratitude you might have for this state, letting yourself fully digest and absorb it.

PART 3
CLEANSING PROTOCOL

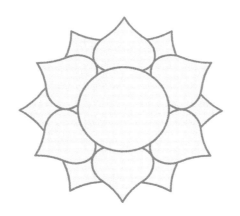

Chapter 7
The Preparation Phase

"Flow is what navigates us through life — not concepts, not ideas, not what we should or shouldn't do, not what's right or wrong. Over time, what we come to see is that flow is always amazing. It is the expression of unity, it directs our existence in ways that are healing and loving and it brings things together in ways we couldn't imagine."

— *Adyashanti, The End of Your World*

Preparation Phase - 4 Days

Diet and Herbs:
- Eat a diet that is low-fat, whole foods, and seasonal. (See specifics that follow.)
- Drink fresh squeezed vegetable and fruit juices, especially apple juice and green vegetable juices. Fresh is best, but Odwalla and Naked brands work, too.
- Eat lots of vegetables to scrub the intestinal lining. Cooked vegetables are easiest to digest. Eat a portion of Beet Liver Cleanser (page 165) with meals.
- Take a Liver Flush Smoothie (page 145) once during Preparation Phase.
- Start your herbal regimen on day 1 of the Preparation Phase, if choosing to take any supplemental herbs.
- Balance your blood sugar levels by including fiber and protein (vegetables, whole grains, legumes) in your meals, and by eating enough at each meal to last until the next meal.
- Continue taking all medications.

Stress Management:
- Practice 10-15+ minutes of yoga, meditation, pranayama or any combination of these, each morning before breakfast, or whenever you can work it into your schedule.

Self-Care:
- Take some extra time for yourself in whatever way feels most relaxing to you. Some ideas are walking in nature, hot baths, extra meditation or prayer time, or extra sleep.
- Plan to cook more than usual during the Preparation Phase. Because the diet does not include any oils with meals, it may be difficult to eat out.

Welcome to the first phase of the cleanse! Hopefully you have gone shopping, familiarized yourself with the basic protocol outlined in Chapter 3 and looked at the stress management and self care practices in Chapters 5 and 6. We now get to put it into action!

The purpose of the Preparation Phase is to prepare the body for the deeper detoxification that happens during the Purification Phase. We move to a low-fat, cleaner diet. This is a gentle segue into eliminating addictive foods.

Additionally, this prepares the inherent detox pathways – the lymph, liver, GI tract and gallbladder – for efficient removal of toxins. By removing difficult-to-digest foods, like heavy meat, dairy and gluten, the digestive system and detox organs are freed up to focus on metabolizing toxins. We add foods such as apples, leafy greens and beets to support healthy liver, gallbladder and lymphatic functioning. We will further prepare the liver for the cleanse with a liver flush. You will also introduce stress management practices into your day such as yoga, pranayama and meditation that was described in the previous chapters.

It is important to note that this is a therapeutic diet, intended to support the cleansing process. It is not meant as a long-term sustainable diet. Some types, especially vata-dominant people benefit from generous fats in their diet and would become more out of balance by following this longer than the cleansing period.

FOOD AND MENUS FOR THE PREPARATION PHASE

Over the next four days, you will eat a low-fat, whole foods diet. Eat in-season as much as possible. The intention in this phase is to eat easy-to-digest lighter foods so that our digestive organs and the liver are primed for the Purification Phase. In many cases, you will start detoxifying during these four days as you eliminate the difficult foods from your body.

Try to stick to three meals per day, at least three hours apart. However, it is important to keep the blood sugar stable. Including fiber and protein (vegetables, beans, whole grains, legumes) in your meals will help keep blood sugar levels steady. If you feel it is a strain to eat only three times per day, add a fourth meal and make sure your meals are big enough to last you to the next one. It may also be helpful to include small amounts of protein, such as lean chicken, some fish (like trout or sardines) or an egg cooked without any oils (hard-boiled, soft, poached) to your midday meal. If you find you are hungry

and can't make it to the next meal, have a snack, such as an apple and seeds, avocado on rice crackers or a green veggie smoothie. This, however, may be an indication that blood sugar is unstable and you may benefit from taking a Gymnema Sylvestre supplement like "Sweet Ease" or "Sugar Destroyer." (See page 95)

Eat your dinner meal early and try to close the kitchen by 7 pm so that you have a long fasting period from your dinner meal to breakfast the next day. This will help the body move into fat-metabolism.

To optimize digestion, eat in a relaxed setting. Take three deep breaths into the belly before your meal, relaxing any tension in the body. Smell your food, say thanks. Eat with awareness, really tasting, feeling and noticing the experience of eating.

Have your biggest meal at midday. Our digestive fire is strongest between 10am and 2pm, so it is best to eat your largest meal at lunchtime. Dinner should be light and easy to digest. Soups and stews are ideal. One simple way of ensuring a satisfying lunch, especially if you are away at work all day, is to make enough at dinner to have leftovers for the next day. By adding some avocado, seeds and/or a grated beet salad (made ahead of time) you will have a complete meal that will keep blood sugar levels steady and sustain energy all day. Be sure to warm your food before lunch, and to never eat food cold or straight from the refrigerator. This dampens digestive fire, resulting in poor digestion and assimilation.

Keep it low in fat. We want the liver to be ready to metabolize the toxins that will begin to be mobilized out of the deeper tissues. By eating less fat during this cleanse, you are giving your liver a much-needed rest so that it can focus on metabolizing toxins and more efficiently burn fat in the future. Avocados and seeds are acceptable fat-rich foods to eat during the Preparation and Rebuilding Phases, however meals and snacks will be made without the use of other fats, such as oils. (The only exception is that ghee can be used in preparing the kitchari for those with vata tendencies. (See pages 101 - 102 for individualizing your cleanse based on your constitution.) Other foods to avoid during the cleanse are listed in the "Foods to Avoid" section that follows. Read the list and take some time to remove these foods from your pantry, if having them around will be difficult for you. In this case, it is important to get support from your partner, spouse or others living with you.

> *Please note that eating a no-fat or extremely low-fat diet long term is not recommended. Our bodies need fat to absorb essential fat-soluble vitamins such as Vitamins A and D. Fat is an excellent source of long, steady burning fuel for our bodies and it is what humans are meant to use for energy and nourishment. Today, we have become reliant on utilizing sugar for energy production, because sugar is so prevalent in our diets. However, sugar burns quickly, leaving our bodies needing more fuel, which means eating again, most likely before the previous meal has been fully digested. Our bodies no longer know how to use fat for fuel, so we are storing it away instead, while being hungry for more fuel.*

FOODS TO EAT DURING THE PREPARATION PHASE

Veggies and Fruit - Focus on non-starchy vegetables, especially those that are green. Choose those that are in season and fresh. Try to have a green smoothie, juice or soup each day during the Preparation Phase. Some of the most beneficial veggies and fruits are:
- **Leafy greens** – This includes spinach, chard, kale, collards, dandelion greens, beet greens, cilantro and parsley. Green veggies are helpful to scrub the intestinal lining and prepare the body for the deeper removal of toxins that will happen in the Purification Phase, so include plenty into your diet at this time. Cilantro and parsley also support removal of heavy metal toxins.
- **Beets** - Try to eat a serving of raw beets everyday. The Beet Liver Cleanser on page 165 is recommended, because raw beets are extremely beneficial for the liver

and they encourage bile production. Having a little with each meal can improve digestion. Cooked beets also support healthy elimination.

- **Apples** – Apples and fresh pressed apple juice support removal of heavy metals, clean the GI tract, regulate bowel function, stimulate bile production and support the liver. Include plenty of these into your diet during your cleanse.
- **Avocado** - Because we are not cooking with oils during the cleansing period, you may find that you need to include some avocado into your meals in order to satisfy your hunger until your next meal. Vata-type people tend to need more fat. Signs that you may need more fat include dry skin, dry constipation and feeling hungry 1-2 hours after eating.

Whole Grains - Focus on gluten-free whole grains such as:

- **Rice** – White rice is easiest to digest and would traditionally be used in an Ayurvedic cleanse, but it is not recommended in cases of diabetes, high blood sugar or Candida yeast overgrowth. Brown, pink, wild, and all other types of rice can be used as well. Rice with the husk on (all rice except white) should ideally be soaked at least six hours or overnight, then drained and cooked in fresh water. The soaking process breaks down phytic acid contained in the husk, which is difficult to digest and blocks absorption of some beneficial nutrients. (See page 206 for more on cooking grains.)
- **Millet** – Millet is easy to digest, has a heating quality and is anti-fungal.
- **Quinoa** – Technically a seed, quinoa is high in protein.
- **Buckwheat** – Excellent for blood sugar regulation, buckwheat is especially good for kapha
- **Amaranth** – Also technically a seed. Amaranth offers a sticky, heavy quality that benefits vata-types.
- **Oats** – Be sure to find gluten free oats; oats are naturally gluten free but are often contaminated when processed on equipment shared with wheat.
- **Rice pasta, rice cakes and rice crackers** made from brown rice (not "rice flour") are okay in moderation.

Beans -These are a good source of lean protein during cleansing, as well as providing plenty of fiber to encourage healthy elimination. This includes black beans, pinto beans, adzuki beans, garbanzo beans (chickpeas), lentils (red, green, black, etc.) and split peas. You can also start eating the split mung beans at this time as well. If you have trouble digesting beans, stick with the smaller beans (lentils, adzuki, split mung) as they will be easier to digest. Large beans, such as garbanzo, are much harder to digest. You will find plenty of recipes using beans in the back of this book.

Soups - Because of their soothing, lubricating nature and ease of digestibility, soups of all kinds are helpful. You will find plenty of soup recipes in the recipe section.

Seeds - These are a good source of protein and fiber. They will also provide some healthy fat while you are not using oils in your cooking. Some good seeds to include are flax, pumpkin, sunflower, sesame, chia and hemp.

Extra Protein, Optional - If you feel you need more protein to keep blood sugar levels steady and/or to satisfy your hunger until the next meal, you can include small amounts of low-fat meat, such as lean chicken or turkey, fish, such as trout and sardines, or a hard-boiled egg.

Spices - Most spices are good because they stimulate digestion, so allow yourself to experiment with different spices in the recipes, including the kitchari. Avoid spices that are excessively hot, such as cayenne. Some especially beneficial spices are:
- **Fresh ginger** – Balancing to all body types, fresh ginger is very beneficial to the digestive tract and helps relieve gas and bloating while stimulating digestive fire.
- **Asafoetida or hing** - This spice is especially beneficial for making beans more digestible.
- **Cardamom** - Helpful for diarrhea, this spice is very soothing to pitta-types.
- **Fennel seeds** - Use fennel seeds to dispel gas and bloating. Good for all types.

Beverages - During the two week cleansing period you will be drinking more liquids than usual. The following are ideal beverages for cleansing:
- **Lots of warm water** - Sipping warm water throughout the day (ideally every 10 minutes) will help the detoxification process by opening and moving the lymphatic system. Try taking a thermos of hot water with you if you are at work or on the go. Plan to drink at least half of your body weight in ounces of water each day.
- **Freshly squeezed apple juice** - Apples have a cleansing effect on the liver and lymph. It is best to have them on an empty stomach as the enzymes and acids in the fruit will help cleanse the lymphatic tissue. Fruit digests quickly, in about 30 minutes or so; if eaten after other foods, the digestion process is slowed and the sugars can begin to ferment, causing gas and bloating.
- **Digestive teas** - Have a digestive tea 10-30 minutes before your meal, a little with the meal, and a few sips afterwards. See page 144 for recipes.
- **Green smoothies and juices** - Lots of vegetables are beneficial during the Preparation Phase because they help scrub the intestinal lining, preparing it for the deeper removal of toxins that will happen during the Purification Phase. See pages 147, 149 and 201 for green drink recipes. You can choose from raw or cooked smoothies, depending on your constitution and what imbalances you are currently experiencing. See pages 101 - 102 for support in individualizing your cleanse according to your constitution.
- **The Liver Flush Smoothie** - Drink a Liver Flush Smoothie one time during the Preparation

Phase. (See page 145 for recipe.) Take between meals or on an empty stomach.

- **Tulsi (holy basil) tea** - Tulsi is a calming herb that supports the nervous system and may promote better sleep. It also has a wonderful fruity taste. There are more and more tulsi teas being offered in bagged form - we like Organic India, particularly their Rose and Masala Chai teas.

FOODS TO AVOID DURING ALL PHASES

- **Wheat and gluten** - Including wheat, barley, rye, couscous, durum, kamut, einkorn, spelt, semolina, triticale, malt, bulgur, wheat bran, wheat germ, wheat starch. Because it is hard to digest, avoid all gluten-containing foods.
- **Bread and yeasted foods** - Including gluten free breads, yeasted flat bread, etc.
- **Flour products** - Such as pasta and crackers, although some simple rice pasta or rice crackers are fine in moderation during the Preparation and Rebuilding phases.
- **Dairy** - Such as butter, yogurt, cheese, milk, lactose, etc. Ghee is acceptable, as it does not contain any of the animal proteins, lactose or casein, and is an important part of the Purification Phase. Fresh yogurt is okay in moderation during the Preparation and Rebuilding Phases.
- **Red meat** - Because it is too heavy and is a building food, not a cleansing food.
- **Fish and shellfish** - Except small amounts of fresh trout, sardines, or salmon if needing extra protein.
- **Nuts and peanuts** - These are too difficult to digest and many types of nuts contain mold.
- **Table salt** - Use only high mineral sea salt and use in moderation, according to constitutional type. Kapha- and pitta-predominant types do better with less salt, while vata types can have a little more.
- **Sweeteners** - Avoid all sweeteners in general, although a little raw honey or stevia is okay during the Preparation and Rebuilding Phases.
- **Caffeine** - A little green tea is okay during your cleanse, but avoid black tea and coffee, including decaf. Coffee in particular is extremely acidic so is not ideal for cleansing.
- **Oils** - Avoid using oils during the Preparation and Purification Phases, although adding some oils back to the diet during the Rebuilding Phase may be important, particularly for vata-predominant types. See pages 101 - 102 for more information regarding how to individualize your cleanse to learn more about oils and constitution types.
- **Cold foods straight from the refrigerator** - Because they will weaken digestive fire and slow digestion.
- **Leftovers more than 24 hours old** - Foods after the first day tend to lose their life-force and begin to break down, which can cause the growth of bacteria.
- **Cold, iced, carbonated drinks** - Because they will weaken digestive fire and slow digestion, as well as aggravating vata.

- **Deep fried foods** - Because they are heavy to digest and contain a lot of fat and oils.
- **Fermented foods like pickles, soy sauce, alcohol** - A little live sauerkraut is okay, and is a valuable part of the Rebuilding Phase, but other fermented foods can become very sharp and aggravate pitta.
- **Frozen foods** - Focus instead on fresh foods that contain life-force energy.
- **Excessively spicy foods** - These will aggravate the tender lining of the intestinal tract and aggravate pitta. They can also cause heartburn and acid reflux.

HERBS FOR CLEANSING

Having done this cleanse successfully many times without the use of herbs, we want to emphasize that they are optional. It is the diet, ghee protocol and lifestyle choices that are the key ingredients to a successful cleanse. We do, however, highly recommend taking the herbal formula triphala beginning with the Rebuilding Phase and continuing for another three weeks after the cleanse. That said, depending on your current state it may be very supportive and enhancing to add other herbs to your protocol. Because these herbs might not be found in your local health food store, you may want to order your herbal supplements ahead of time to ensure they arrive in time for your home cleanse. At the end of this section is a list of Ayurvedic herb vendors we like.

The following is a brief description of the herbs, their main action in facilitating the cleanse and some key points to help you decide if this herb might be right for you as a supplement during the cleanse. Please note, an Ayurvedic practitioner can more accurately recommend the best herbs for your constitution and current state. If you are taking medication, continue to take them as usual throughout the cleanse. It is advised to check with your physician for any known contraindications. It is always okay to discontinue taking an herb at any time during the cleanse if you are concerned with its effect in any way.

- **Gymnema sylvestre** (*gurmar*): Usually combined in a formula, such as "Sweet Ease" or "Sugar Destroyer," this herb helps to slow down sugar absorption and curb cravings for the sweet taste. If you tend to have high blood sugar and/or a sweet tooth, this is a good herb to consider. Take one capsule prior to each meal. You can take this through all phases of the cleanse and for an additional two weeks afterwards.

- **Trikatu:** This is a formula combining "three hots," which are ginger, black pepper, and long pepper (*pippali*). This is a traditional formula to awaken digestion and increase the capacity to digest toxins. It is a rejuvenative for the lung tissue and is often taken during a cold. Consider this herb when digestion is weak. It is contraindicated when there is excess pitta and hyperacidity. In these cases see "Cool Digest" below. Take one capsule prior to each meal. You can take this through all phases of the cleanse and for an additional two weeks afterwards.

- **Cool Digest or Pitta Digest**: These formulas are alternatives to trikatu when there is excess pitta in the system. They stimulate digestion without increasing heat or aggravating pitta. Ingredients vary and often combine triphala and trikatu with some cooling herbs, such as vidanga, neem, guduchi, kutaja and/or avipatikar. Consider adding this herb combination if digestion is weak and you have a pitta constitution, particularly if you have a tendency toward heartburn or acid reflux. Take one capsule prior to each meal. You can take this through all phases of the cleanse and for an additional two weeks afterwards.

- **Beet Cleanse**: This can be added to your protocol to increase bile production and encourage the movement of bile flow, thereby decreasing congestion in the liver, gallbladder and ducts. This has a similar action to the Beet Liver Cleanser (see page 165). It is useful for those who don't like to eat beets and yet still want to support this aspect of cleansing. Take one capsule prior to each meal. You can take this through all phases of the cleanse and for an additional two weeks afterwards.

- **Manjishta**: The main attribute of this herb is that it is a powerful blood cleanser. It is cooling in nature and has an amazing capacity to clear the blood and lymph of excess heat, inflammation and toxins. Because of this, it has a positive effect on the skin tissue and helps clear rashes, acne, eczema, psoriasis, etc. It has decongestant properties for the liver and kidneys. If you tend to have skin rashes, swelling (especially before menstruation), pervasive fatigue or allergies, this is a good herb to consider. Take one capsule after each meal. You can take this through all phases of the cleanse and for an additional two weeks afterwards.

- **Turmeric**: The "golden girl" of herbs, turmeric has many wonderful attributes and uses. In the context of this cleanse, it is used to heal the walls of the intestinal tract. It does this by pulling excess mucous from the digestive tract and repairing and soothing any damage from inflammation. It strengthens digestion and improves the microbiome of the gut. It also increases blood flow to the liver and helps increase bile flow. Consider turmeric as a supplement if you are not using generous amounts of turmeric in your kitchari meals during the Purification Phase, or if you suffer from inflammation. Take one capsule after each meal. You can take this through all phases of the cleanse and for an additional two weeks afterwards.

- **Bhumiamalaki**: A main component to the formulas Liver Repair, Liver Assist and Liver Support. These herbal formulas support the liver in detoxification and rejuvenation. Bhumi-amalaki has an affinity for the liver and can improve its function while clearing inflammation. It promotes the flow of bile and helps prevent gallstones. Recommended when the liver has been compromised through excessive alcohol or drug use and toxic exposure and with signs of excess pitta, such as skin conditions and inflammation. Take one capsule after each meal. You can take this through all phases of the cleanse and for an additional two weeks afterwards.

- **Triphala**: Triphala is an ancient and very popular formula from Ayurveda. It is made up of three dried fruits: amalaki, bibhitaki and haritaki. It is a digestive tonic and supports healthy elimination. Although it has a mild laxative effect, it does not create dependency. It is balancing to all three doshas and is cleansing and rejuvenating to all tissues in the body. Triphala is also naturally very high in Vitamin C. Take one to two capsules about an hour before bedtime or one to two capsules in the morning, about an hour before breakfast. We recommend starting this herb during the Rebuilding Phase and then continuing to take it for another three weeks. It can also be taken during the other phases if constipation arises and as a substitute for castor oil when indicated.

- **Castor oil**: Used internally as a strong laxative during the cleanse, it has the ability to completely flush the large intestine. Because it is an emollient, it simultaneously soothes the lining of the colon. Castor oil has been used internally in Ayurveda for thousands of years. Be sure to find a castor oil that is hexane-free or organic.

- **Ghee**: In the context of the cleanse, we are using ghee as a chelator to pull the fat-soluble toxins out of the cells. However, it has some wonderfully healing attributes, as well. Free of the milk proteins that are difficult to digest, it helps the body absorb nutrients. Ghee has a unique ability to penetrate the lipid bilayer of the cells in the gut, skin, heart and arteries and restore lubrication and lymphatic movement. It is high in vitamin A and D, as well as conjugated linolenic acid (CLA.) CLA is involved in the body's ability to regulate fat. Ghee is also high in butyric acid. This substance feeds the good bacteria in the gut, which are crucial for good digestion, strong immunity, and stable moods. Ghee contains no lactose or casein if properly clarified. For more information on how you will be using ghee, see page 107.

- **Dashamula**: This is an ancient formula composed of ten roots. In the context of the cleanse, it is used for making the "tea" that goes in the basti (enema) formula. This helps to cleanse and tone the large intestine. It can also be taken internally as a tea to soothe vata imbalances and relieve pain. It is especially helpful for headaches.

- **Digestive Teas**: Try some of the herbal blends on page 144 in the Recipes section, or feel free to combine some of the herbs to create your own favorite digestive tea.

- **Abhyanga Oils**: These are herbal oils used for self-massage during the cleanse. We commonly use mahanarayan oil, which is good for all constitutions. It is an ancient formula that has many healing herbs in a sesame oil base. The oil acts as a delivery mechanism so that the herbs can penetrate deeper into the tissues. The oil is soothing and grounding to the nervous system and acts as a protective buffer. However, any tri-doshic ayurvedic blend is also appropriate for self-abhyanga. If you know your particular doshic makeup, you can use a blend specific for your constitution. It is best to use the herbal blended oils, but it is also okay to use plain organic sesame oil or a combination of sesame with organic sunflower, almond or coconut oil. Sesame is particularly great during cleansing as its heavy, nourishing properties help support the nervous system. See pages 81 - 83 for more information on body oils.

Resources for Buying Herbs, Ghee and Oil

- lifespa.com
- banyanbotanicals.com
- tattvaherbs.com
- floracopeia.com
- shaktiveda.com
- saradausa.com
- ayurveda.com
- ancientorganics.com

SAMPLE MENUS FOR THE PREPARATION PHASE

Sample Day 1:
- *Upon Rising*: Big glass of warm water
- *Before breakfast (10-15 Minutes)*: Digestive tea or 8 oz. fresh pressed apple juice, pre-meal supplements
- *Breakfast*: Green smoothie and/or Creamy Rice Cereal with cooked fruit and seeds.
- *Before Lunch (10-15 Minutes)*: Digestive Tea and pre-meal supplements
- *Lunch*:
    - Vegetarian: Beet Liver Cleanser, Black Beans with Avocado & Corn
    - More Protein: Beet Liver Cleanser, Baked Rainbow Trout, steamed vegetables and brown rice with Creamy Oil-Free Dressing
- *Before Dinner (10-15 Minutes)*: Digestive Tea and pre-meal supplements
- *Dinner*: Beet Liver Cleanser, Gingery Butternut Apple Soup with rice crackers

Sample Day 2:
- *Upon Rising*: Big glass of warm water
- *Before breakfast (10-15 Minutes)*: Digestive tea, pre-meal supplements
- *Breakfast*: 8 oz apple juice (drink first), Green smoothie and/or Chia Cereal
- *Before Lunch (10-15 Minutes)*: Digestive Tea and pre-meal supplements
- *Lunch*:
    - Vegetarian: Beet Liver Cleanser, Garlicky Millet Mash, and Green smoothie
    - More Protein: Beet Liver Cleanser, Sardines with Shaved Fennel, quinoa with coconut aminos or Bragg's
- *Before Dinner (10-15 Minutes)*: Digestive Tea and pre-meal supplements
- *Dinner*: Blended Black Bean Soup with cilantro and lime juice, Beet Liver Cleanser

A Note About Organic Foods

Obviously, a big part of the cleansing process is removing toxins from the body. Therefore, during your two week cleanse, you want to focus on foods that have the lowest toxin load. While you don't have to source everything certified organic, there are some foods that are higher in pesticide residues than others, and some foods that have questionable origins when raised conventionally. The following is a list of some of the foods you want to consider sourcing organically.

Produce – When it comes to fresh produce, pesticide residues are the main concern. Some crops, such as onions and garlic, contain little or no residues because pests do not care for them. A thick peel protects others, such as bananas, so the edible part contains little or no residue. However, some fruits and vegetables are a prime target for pests and have to be heavily treated in order to be market-worthy. The Environmental Working Group provides an up-to-date list each year of the "Dirty Dozen" and "Clean 15" so consumers are aware of which crops should be sourced organically and which don't matter. Go to http://www.ewg.org/ to find out more. Most of all, remember that fresh food is best, so even if you cannot find organic produce where you live, be sure to still include plenty of fresh fruits and vegetables into your cleanse.

Animal foods – Modern farming methods cause some concern for what kind of meat is making its way to your plate. Antibiotics given to animals that transfer to the consumer, inhumane treatment and genetically modified feed that causes inflammation are all real issues today. While the purpose of this book is not to tout any agenda, it is important that we become aware of what we are eating, particularly when the food in question was previously walking and breathing. This is an important point in Ayurvedic medicine: you are what you eat and digest. When we raise a chicken to grow in 20 days the size it should grow in 20 weeks, we are aging our body years for every week.

Try to source animal products organically whenever possible. (This includes meat, eggs and dairy, although only some of these will be eaten during the cleansing period.) Local is also a great way to go – if you have met your farmer and have seen where your food comes from, that is more valuable than any third-party seal of approval. If you are unable to find organic, look for other signs that your food is clean, such as "raised without antibiotics" or "humanely raised and handled." This is a vast subject that we cannot fully cover in this book, but there are plenty of good books on the market today covering this issue.

Soy products – Because the majority of soy being grown today is genetically modified, it is important to find soy products that are organic. Ayurveda is clear on this issue: when we alter nature's genes, we are altering our own genes.

SAMPLE DAILY ROUTINE FOR CLEANSING

1. Rise with the sun, or at around 6 AM.
2. Drink a large glass of warm or room temperature water.
3. Spend 10+ minutes practicing yoga, meditation and breathing techniques.
4. Apply oil to skin and allow to absorb for at least 10 minutes.
5. Shower or bathe.
6. Eat breakfast when hungry, in a relaxed manner.
7. Have lunch mid-day, spending time relaxing and enjoying your food. This should be your largest meal.
8. Walk a little outside in the fresh air.
9. Eat dinner early and let it be light and simple, such as a soup or veggie stew. Close the kitchen by 7pm.
10. Spend another 10 minutes before bed winding down. Try a few simple yoga poses like forward bend, supported shoulder bridge or legs up the wall, meditation, breathing practices, walking or simply relaxing.
11. Turn lights out by 10 pm.

INDIVIDUALIZING YOUR CLEANSE BASED ON YOUR MINDBODY TYPE

Based on your results from the assessment from Chapter 2, you can begin to get a sense of your predominant dosha(s) and where you are most out of balance. By bringing extra awareness to your imbalanced dosha during and after the cleansing period, you can begin to bring your body back to its natural center. The following are ways you can individualize your cleanse to address an imbalance you may be experiencing.

For vata tendency:
- Adjust your cleanse by using some ghee in your kitchari or mung soup.
- Use copious amounts of external oil for your self-massage.
- Pare down your schedule as much as possible.
- Stay warm.
- If using a digestive herb before meals, use trikatu or a vata-specific digestive formula.
- Drink digestive teas using ginger, fennel, tulsi and/or licorice.

- Add limes, coconut and/or fresh ginger to kitchari/mung meal.
- If needed, eat four small meals each day.
- Try the High Protein Kitchari (page 234) if feeling weak or hungry.

For pitta tendency:
- If using a pre-meal digestive herbal formula, use Cool Digest, Pitta Digest or a similar pitta-pacifying combination.
- Drink a digestive tea that has equal parts cumin, coriander and fennel with a little cardamom.
- Add coconut and/or cilantro to kitchari/mung meal.
- Make sure to eat all meals and use liver-supporting herbs.
- If using a sauna, don't stay in longer than 15 minutes.
- Practice surrendering to the process.
- Try the High Protein Kitchari (page 234) if feeling hungry between meals.

For kapha tendency:
- If using a pre-meal digestive herbal formula, use trikatu. (This may be found under names such as Warm Digest or Kapha Digest.)
- Add a digestive tea using cumin, coriander, fennel, cardamom, clove and/or cinnamon. Ginger and tulsi are also good on their own or to add to your tea.
- Add plenty of spices to kitchari/mung soup – all spices are good for pacifying kapha.
- Keep moving during the cleanse: walking or yoga are especially helpful. Get some movement every day.

If you are not sure about your constitution, which dosha is most out of balance, or feel equally all three, then follow the general guidelines, but feel free to experiment with the adjustments above depending on how you are feeling that particular day.

Preparation Phase Check List:

☐ Low fat, whole foods diet ☐ Beets
☐ Optional herbs ☐ Lots of vegetables (especially green)
☐ Liver flush smoothie ☐ Stress management: yoga, pranayama, meditation
☐ Apples ☐ Self care: extra rest and relaxation

Chapter 8
The Purification Phase

"If you 'pinch an inch' around your waist, the fat you are squeezing between your fingers is not the same as it was last month. Your adipose tissues (fat cells) fill up with fat and empty out constantly, so that all of it is exchanged every three weeks. You acquire a new stomach lining every five days (the innermost layer of stomach cells is exchanged in a matter of minutes as you digest food). Your skin is new every five weeks."

– Deepak Chopra, Perfect Health

Purification Phase - 7-8 Days

Diet and Herbs:
- Eat a primarily kitchari diet. (See pages 105 - 107 for meal options and pages 228 - 237 for recipes.)
- Take melted ghee each morning on an empty stomach. (See page 107 for schedule). Wait until you feel hunger before eating breakfast (at least 15 minutes).
- Drink the purgative on Day 7 of the Purification Phase. If possible, take this between 10am and 2pm on an empty stomach, or at least 2 hours after eating.
- Administer an enema on Day 8 (optional).
- Continue taking all medications.
- Continue taking any herbs for the cleanse.
- Stop taking any supplements that are not part of the cleanse, if you feel you can go without them. If you normally take fish, flax or borage oil capsules and feel you cannot go without them, take them with the morning ghee.

Stress Management:
- Practice 10-15+ minutes of pranayama, yoga and/or meditation daily.

Self-Care:
- Include a self-oil massage before a hot bath, shower or sauna daily.

* Schedule Days 7 and 8 of the Purification Phase at a time when you can be at home relaxing because of the purgative and basti on these days.

Welcome to the Purification Phase, the main part of your cleanse! For some of you, the Preparation Phase may have been challenging. Depending on your normal diet, you may have been exploring a whole new way of eating. You have been preparing your body, simplifying your diet, adding herbs and/or certain foods and learning stress management practices. Take a moment to acknowledge what you have already accomplished. You are now ready for the next phase of the journey. The experience will be unique to you, but in this chapter, we provide some general landmarks to look for

that may help you feel confident that you are on the right road. These are found in the "What to Expect Day by Day" section of this chapter.

This 7 - 8 day Purification Phase helps you enter fat metabolism mode, pulls toxins from deep within your tissues and moves the toxins to your digestive system for removal. This phase also balances blood sugar (and thus mood and energy), improves digestion, and opens your detox channels. Each morning for seven days you will drink increasing amounts of melted ghee. The seven day time frame is important because it takes seven days to reach and saturate each of the seven tissue systems of the body. However, do not take ghee for more than seven days, as this will exceed the body's ability to use it productively. Along with this very easy-to-digest diet and ghee, you will be including oil self-massage and stress management practices each day.

On the seventh day, you will be taking a purgative (a strong laxative).

On the eighth day, you will have the option of administering a basti (an herbal water and sesame oil enema).

FOOD & MENUS DURING THE PURIFICATION PHASE

The main thing to remember when eating during the Purification Phase is that you want your food to be light and easy to digest. During the 7-8 day Purification Phase, you will be eating kitchari (split mung beans with a gluten-free grain, such as rice or quinoa) as your main food. You can make the split mung beans as a soup and have the grain served separately, or make it together in one dish, which is the traditional preparation method for kitchari. (See pages 231 - 237 for several different kitchari recipes.)

Just as in the Preparation Phase, you want to avoid heavy foods, difficult-to-digest foods, sugar, alcohol and caffeine. In addition, you want to greatly reduce pungent (spicy) foods, salt and fermented foods. We are focusing on

a *sattvic* diet, one that promotes a clear and peaceful mind, so we are choosing foods with a gentle quality. The diet can be augmented with steamed or baked veggies, small mounts of cooked fruit and lean protein as needed. Avoid fats and oils (including avocados and nuts). The exception to this is the ghee you will be taking each morning and small amounts of ghee in kitchari for vata-types. (See pages 101 - 102 for tips on individualizing your cleanse.) Continue drinking digestive teas and sip plenty of warm to hot water throughout the day.

Foods to Eat During the Purification Phase:
- Split mung beans
- Light, whole grains, such as rice or quinoa
- Vegetables – Most are good, but avoid Cruciferous veggies (broccoli, cabbage, kale, collards), Alliums (onions, garlic, leeks) and Nightshades (potatoes, tomatoes, peppers, and eggplant); also avoid avocado
- Fruit – Cooked is easiest to digest; this can be eaten on its own or added to a cooked grain cereal, such as rice farina, for breakfast
- Plenty of spices – Most are good, but avoid excessively pungent ones, such as cayenne
- Small amounts of seeds, if needed for protein and/or blood sugar balance
- Condiments, such as fresh squeezed lemon or lime, cilantro, parsley, and unsweetened shredded coconut
- Plenty of digestive teas and warm water

It is important to keep blood sugar stable. Aim for three meals per day; eat enough to get you to the next meal, preferably without snacking. Because we are all working with different body types and conditions, please modify this diet when needed. In general, as the morning ghee intake increases, blood sugar will stabilize and it will be easier to go for longer periods between meals. However, until that happens, you can try modifying in any of the ways listed below. Please rest assured that using these modifications will not hamper your cleanse. There is no need to push through hunger. Being comfortable and keeping stress low is more important for the process. Remember that your body is better able to release toxins when the mindbody is at ease and when blood sugar is stable.

Modifications include:

- *Add small amounts of lean protein to a meal.* If you feel the fuel from your mung bean meal is not getting you to the next meal without hunger in between, try the High Protein Kitchari (page 234) or add small amounts of white chicken, freshwater fish or a poached or boiled egg to your kitchari. Freshwater fish, such as trout, tends to be lower in fat.
- *Add some ghee to your mung beans.* If you have a vata constitution or are currently vata-imbalanced, it may be helpful to cook your mung beans with some ghee (a tablespoon is plenty).
- *Add a fourth meal.* Be sure to space your meals at least three hours apart to allow for proper digestion and to encourage the body to begin utilizing its fat stores.

Why Kitchari?

Kitchari is a mixture of split mung beans and rice. It is the traditional dietary base for panchakarma for several reasons.

Firstly, it is easy to digest. It doesn't tax the digestive system, therefore freeing up digestive organs to work on breaking down and getting rid of toxins.

Secondly, while it is light, it is incredibly nourishing, meeting our nutritional needs while balancing all three doshas: vata, pitta and kapha.

In addition, the astringent quality of the mung beans helps to pull ama out of the body. The spices typically present in kitchari, such as turmeric and cumin, are also detoxifying and help clear excess mucous off intestinal walls.

Finally, the fiber content in kitchari binds to the toxic substances that are pulled into the gastrointestinal tract, making it easier to be evacuated from the body.

Getting a little tired of mung beans?

Variations include:
- *Have a gluten-free grain for your breakfast meal.* Sometimes mung beans do not seem appetizing in the morning. Whenever you like, you can have warm cereal such as oats, millet, quinoa or rice for your morning meal. It is also okay to cook fruit into it, such as apples, pears or berries.
- *Try a mung soup.* Soup is easier to re-heat and it is much easier to add a variety of veggies into. A root veggie with a green veggie is a nice mix, such as spinach and carrots, green beans and beets or collards and yams.
- *Have a sweet potato or stewed apple dessert to satisfy a sweet craving.* See our simple recipes for Cinnamon Apples & Raisins (page 162) or Baked Yams & Apples (page 168).

Ghee Schedule
For seven days you will be taking ghee immediately after rising each morning. (See page 108 for vegan/alternative options.) The amount you should take is individual and the chart that follows gives suggested ranges. Work within the comfort of your body and gradually work up to your limit over the seven days. Don't push beyond tolerance! For instance, feeling a little nauseated after ghee intake is normal, but if it doesn't dissipate after an hour, you probably took too much and can ease back a little the next day. If you feel the cleanse is too intense in any way, you can always ease back on ghee intake. Only increase daily dosage if you are tolerating it. If you experience loose or painful stools or nausea that lasts more than 10 minutes, then do not increase the dose of ghee the next morning. Stay at the current dose or slightly lower until you are comfortable, and then increase.

Ghee should be taken first thing in the morning on an empty stomach. This signals to the body that it will be burning fat for fuel. It may be helpful to eat a small piece of raw ginger or drink a little ginger tea right before or after the ghee intake. A small amount of unsweetened soy, almond or rice milk right after ghee really cuts the taste as well, or try holding your nose while drinking the ghee. Wait until hunger returns before eating breakfast, at least 15 minutes after taking the ghee.

Day 1:	1 - 2 tsp
Day 2:	2 - 4 tsp
Day 3:	4 - 6 tsp
Day 4:	4 - 6 tsp
Day 5:	6 - 8 tsp
Day 6:	6 - 8 tsp
Day 7:	8 - 10 tsp

Purgation
By day seven of the Purification Phase, you have most likely pulled toxins from the deep tissues into the gastrointestinal tract through ghee saturation. Bile produced by the liver attaches to these fats, escorting them into the small intestines through the common bile duct.

The Importance of Ghee

Ghee is clarified butter, in which all the difficult-to-digest animal protein has been removed. You can purchase your ghee at most grocery stores and local health food stores, buy it online, or clarify organic, unsalted butter at home. It's extremely simple - go to page 230 to read the recipe. When properly clarified, ghee contains no lactose and only trace amounts of casein, although some sources say their product is free of casein, as well. Ghee contains butyric acid, which feeds the beneficial gut microbes that keep the damaging microbes in check. The benefits of ghee include promoting optimal assimilation of nutrients, supporting healthy elimination, boosting immunity, balancing moods and supporting hydration.

The ingestion of ghee each morning during the Purification Phase is a unique attribute of the Ayurvedic method of cleansing, known as internal oleation. This protocol actually pulls fat-soluble toxins out of the body. Ghee acts like a cleansing scrub in the body, getting between cells and loosening up the ama (toxic sludge) that has accumulated. Because toxins are fat-soluble, the saturation of ghee outside the cells draws the toxins out of the cells and into the fat. In addition, the high fat content of ghee signals the body to produce large amounts of bile. This helps to flush out the bile ducts that may have become congested and inefficient. Finally, ingesting fat first thing in the morning on an empty stomach puts the body on track to metabolize fat for fuel. This helps blood sugar stability and promotes sustained, even-keeled energy all day. All of these attributes improve the ability to digest fat and the fat-soluble toxins in the future and contributes to long-lasting, positive effects of the Ayurvedic cleanse. **If you are vegan or concerned about the use of ghee, you can alternatively use flax oil or olive oil.** These will effectively pull fat soluble toxins out.

Taking a strong laxative will remove toxins that have accumulated in the small intestine. Because the small intestines are considered the home of the pitta function in the body, this tends to relieve pitta-like organs and qualities as well. The liver and gallbladder are considered pitta organs and are thus relieved of excess heat through this process. Although you will experience loose bowels, this is very different from having diarrhea due to an infection or parasite. In this herbally-induced purgation, the effect will be short term. Once it subsides, you will feel clearer and lighter as toxic wastes have been eliminated from the body.

Purgative Directions
In this home cleanse we suggest using organic castor oil as the purgative.* The dosage varies by body type. 4 - 6 teaspoons are usually adequate to produce a laxative effect. If you have pitta tendencies or a pitta imbalance, stick to the lower dosage.

You can substitute five triphala capsules or two teaspoons of triphala powder for the castor oil purgative. (Equivalent formulas like Life Spa's "Elim 1" or Shakti Veda's "Cleanse Within" are also fine.) This option is for those who have been having a lot of loose stools throughout the cleanse, have concerns regarding their gallbladder, or are just are not willing to take the castor oil.

Purgation (*virechena*) affects the small intestine, which is the home of pitta dosha. It is therefore recommended to take the purgative during the pitta time of day, which is 10 am – 2 pm. Take it on an empty stomach, at least two hours after food. If that time of day won't work for

you, don't worry, do it when you can relax. Take a nice bath after taking the purgative and/or place a hot water bottle on your tummy. Doing something that is relaxing and distracts you is useful, such as watching a mellow movie or reading a book. On your purgation day, keep the diet simple and easy.

Castor Oil Purgative
You will need:
4 - 6 tsp organic or hexane-free castor oil
Juice of an orange or grapefruit
Hot water

Mix castor oil with the orange or grapefruit juice and add a little hot water. (Set aside a wedge of orange or grapefruit for afterwards.) Hold your nose and drink the castor mix, then immediately suck on the orange wedge. Usually, there is a laxative effect one to five hours later. Wait till this wears off before eating again.

You may have several bowel movements during this time and it will most likely get to a liquid state. It is important to stay hydrated. In the case of many bowel movements, you may want to take an electrolyte beverage afterwards. (See recipe on following page.)

Occasionally, some people may not experience a laxative effect from the castor oil. This indicates chronic dryness in the colon. If possible, see an Ayurvedic practitioner on how to work with this. The castor oil will still have a beneficial effect because it begins to add moisture to an overly-dry colon. However, it is important to make sure you have flushed out all of the toxins that have moved to the digestive tract during the cleansing period. If you do not have a laxative effect, drink some warm water, massage castor oil into the abdomen and cover with a small towel. Then, place a hot water bottle on abdomen. Following this, take five triphala capsules. It is also recommended to do the enema (*basti*) the next day.

Optional Enema (*Basti*)

Basti is one of the traditional "five actions" of panchakarma. Bastis are helpful after the cleansing purgative to ensure that everything gets effectively eliminated from the colon. If you experience constipation, a basti on day 8 of the Purification Phase or a series of bastis during the Rebuilding Phase will be especially beneficial. (See page 36 for directions for this enhanced version.) The enema will clear the colon of accumulated toxins, provide nourishment for good bacteria in the colon, and balance the vata dosha.

Enemas should be done in the morning or in the evening on an empty stomach, preferably before breakfast or three hours after eating. If you are planning on doing the herbal enema, it is recommended to do it during vata time, between 2 pm and 6 pm. If you'd rather do it in the morning, you could do it around sunrise. This, again, should be on an empty stomach. Administering it in the bath is relaxing and easy. If you feel weak from the purgation, wait a day before doing the enema. Keep the diet simple and easy to digest, such as a baked yam with sunflower seeds, steamed veggies with rice or veggie soup.

Simple Electrolyte Beverage

You will need:
½ cup fresh squeezed lemon or lime juice
2 cups water
⅛ tsp sea salt
1 - 2 Tablespoons natural sugar or honey

Blend all ingredients together and drink slowly.

Basti Directions

You will need:
1 Tbsp dashamula powder
    (or 2 Tbsp whole root)
1 ½ cups water
½ cup sesame oil

1. Combine dashamula powder or whole root in water and bring to a boil. Lower heat and simmer for 5-7 minutes. Turn off heat and cool to body temperature.
2. Strain the tea and add sesame oil. Mix well and add to enema bag.
3. Follow the directions provided with your enema bag for administering. Once mixture is inserted, try to retain liquid for several minutes. Evacuate when needed.

Tips: It is comfortable to administer the enema in the bathtub. Also, try putting a little bit of sesame oil on the insertion tube. The bath will relax you and the proximity to the toilet is convenient.

SAMPLE MENU FOR THE PURIFICATION PHASE

- *Upon Rising:* Drink melted ghee followed by a little warm water
- *Before breakfast (10-15 minutes):* Digestive tea, pre-meal supplements
- *Breakfast:* Hot Rice Cereal with pumpkin seeds, cooked pears and cardamom
- *Before Lunch (10-15 Minutes):* Digestive Tea and pre-meal supplements
- *Lunch:* Kitchari with steamed veggies
- *Before Dinner (10-15 Minutes):* Digestive Tea and pre-meal supplements
- *Dinner:* Kitchari

Other meal ideas include baked sweet potato with shredded, unsweetened coconut or simply rice with steamed veggies and pumpkin seeds. This is especially welcome in the later part of the Purification Phase when you may need a meal break from mung beans. (See pages 228 - 229 for more Purification Phase meal ideas.)

STRESS MANAGEMENT & SELF-CARE FOR THE PURIFICATION PHASE

Stress management and self-care are most important during this phase. As toxins loosen, so do emotions. By putting in place routines that allow you to sort through these emotions without judging them, you are allowing yourself to also release them. Be sure to place as much priority on these practices as you do on diet.

As outlined in the chart overview at the beginning of this chapter, you will administer a self massage each day, followed by a hot bath with Epsom salts or a sauna. If you don't have a bath or sauna, simply take a hot shower and allow yourself to spend as much time as you need to relax and enjoy it. The heat and oleation (oiling) process further facilitates removal of toxic build up.

Be sure to practice at least 10 or 15 minutes of pranayama and yoga each day. Morning is optimal, but please feel free to do this whenever it is best for your schedule. These practices also help to move toxins through the body to the gastrointestinal tract, where they can then be evacuated. Immediately after your pranayama and yoga practice is an ideal time to sit in meditation or prayer.

Also during this phase, be sure to get to bed early. Much of the liver's cleansing work is done during sleeping hours from 10 pm to 2 am.

WHAT TO EXPECT DAY BY DAY

These are just some common sign posts that may come up on your journey. Of course, each individual will have a unique experience, so don't worry if your experience is different or if you are not experiencing these things at all.

Because each day of the cleanse is associated with cleansing one of the seven body tissues in a particular order, you may have experiences that correspond to detoxing that tissue. For instance on day three, the detoxification occurs in the muscle tissue (*mamsa dhatu*). This may cause muscle aches or fatigue as the toxins are being dislodged from this tissue.

Day 1

Begin the day with 1-2 teaspoons of melted and slightly cooled ghee
Rasa Dhatu, lymphatic tissue
You may feel hungry. If this is the case, try eating four meals on this day. Try to keep the meals spaced at least three hours apart. If you are not able to go three hours without hunger, add a little chicken breast, sardines or a hard-boiled egg to a meal. You may feel tired or have headaches, especially if you are purging caffeine and sugar out of your system. You may notice how much the caffeine and sugar were masking an underlying lack of real energy. Try drinking lots of fluids, especially teas like ginger, licorice, hibiscus and dashamula. You also may experience a small amount of bloating or heaviness. If so, make sure you are drinking digestive teas and add hing to your kitchari. Make sure you are staying warm and keeping out of the wind.

Day 2

Begin the day with 2-4 tsp ghee
Rakta Dhatu, blood/circulation
Again there may be fatigue and weakness, especially as the liver is working hard to process toxins. You may notice sugar cravings crop up. If this comes up, try eating more bitters. The taste of bitter is the anecdote for the sweet taste. Use lots of arugula, dandelion and parsley in your split mung meal. Also, you may need to add the "Sweet Ease" herb, gymnema sylvestre. Many folks will begin to feel stronger emotions at this point. Often irritability, anger and the old stories around these

emotions may come up. Be gentle with yourself. Try to be understanding of these emotions and witness them with compassion. Journal, walk, do yoga, drink cucumber water.

Day 3

Begin the day with 4-6 tsp ghee
Mamsa Dhatu, muscle tissue
Again, emotions may be coming to the surface. Your body and muscles, in particular, may be especially tired on this day. Do gentle exercise, like slow mindful yoga and meditation. Drink lots of fluids.

Day 4

Begin the day with 4-6 tsp ghee
Meda Dhatu, fat tissue
Ghee intake may begin to be more difficult on this day. (Try some tricks like sucking on a lemon or lime wedge, taking ginger tea or taking a shot of unsweetened soy or rice milk before or after your ghee.) However, this is often when fat metabolism sets in. You may find you are more satisfied between meals and that your energy is more even and calm. Again, stay open to the emotions that are surfacing and take notice of your dreams. Try journaling or just sitting with awareness. Enjoy nature.

Day 5

Begin the day with 6-8 tsp ghee
Asthi Dhatu, bone tissue
By day five you may begin to feel lighter and clearer. You may notice heightened senses and a vivid experience of the world. With this increased sensitivity, be mindful of keeping stimulation, activities and socializing to a minimum. Take advantage of this clarity to meditate and take stock of what really matters in your life. Be gentle on yourself. Seek nature, rest and oil your body well. This is a good day for an abhyanga and/or shirodhara treatment.

Day 6

Begin the day with 6-8 tsp ghee
Majja Dhatu, nerve tissue
This day will be similar to day five. You may notice your appetite has gone down. Continue to walk gently through your day and savor this clear seeing. Again, a really good day for Ayurvedic body therapies.

Day 7

Begin the day with 8-10 tsp ghee
Shukra/Artava Dhatu, reproductive tissue – male/female accordingly
Day seven will be your last day for taking ghee in the morning. Eat a small, light meal once you have an appetite again. On this day, you will take a purgative to induce a laxative effect.

Day 8

No ghee today! This day varies, depending on how the purgation went. You may feel light and clear or you may feel tired and vulnerable. It is very soothing to finish your panchakarma with a professional oil massage (abhyanga).

Purification Phase Checklist:
- ☐ Kitchari diet
- ☐ Morning ghee
- ☐ Optional herbs
- ☐ Daily yoga, pranayama and meditation
- ☐ Daily self abhyanga and bath, sauna or shower
- ☐ Regular elimination
- ☐ Purgation on Day 7
- ☐ Basti on Day 8 (optional)

TROUBLESHOOTING

Elimination

Because we are mobilizing toxins during this cleanse, it is important to make sure you eliminate everyday. Kitchari can cause constipation for some people because of its astringent nature. If you experience constipation, be sure to refer to the tips listed below. Healthy elimination varies by constitutional type.

Elimination by Constitutional Type

- Vata - Normal vata elimination happens one time per day, ideally in the first few hours after waking. Stools should be easy to pass and fully formed. Imbalanced stools for vata may be dry, hard, difficult to pass, incomplete, less than once per day and/or many small pebble-like stools, similar to deer pellets.
- Pitta - Normal pitta elimination happens two times per day, usually once just after rising and again after lunch. Pitta-type stools should be fully formed but break apart when flushed. Imbalanced pitta stools are loose, tend toward diarrhea and happen more frequently than twice per day. They may be more yellow or light brown in color and may be accompanied by a burning sensation.
- Kapha - Normal kapha elimination happens once per day, usually just after rising, and is copious. They are fully formed and have little odor. Imbalanced kapha stools tend to be thick, sticky and slow-moving.

Please note that the elimination by constitution type outlined here is an ideal for daily life and not necessarily what happens when we are cleansing. Between the ghee, eating a mono-diet and the elimination of toxins, it is common to experience variations in bowel movements throughout the cleanse.

Constipation

The following are tips you can try in case of constipation.

- Make sure you are drinking enough water. You should be drinking half of your body weight in ounces each day and the water should be warm or hot. Tea made from fresh ginger, or any of the other digestive tea recipes on page 144 can account for some of this water intake, but be sure you are drinking plenty of plain water.

- Add triphala to your cleanse, which you can find at most health food stores. See page 97 for more information on this herb.
- Do at least a little yoga and the three pranayama practices (see pages 78 - 79) everyday to massage the colon. A gentle stomach massage is also helpful during your daily yoga practice.
- Make sure dinner is light and early.
- Try the sipping the Elimination Tea (page 150) throughout the day.
- Add extra fiber. During the Preparation and Rebuilding Phases, eat the Beet Liver Cleanser and a green smoothie every day. During Purification, you can add non-starchy vegetables to your kitchari and/or eat cooked beets.
- Increase your dose of liver supporting herbs.
- Cook prunes into rice cereal for breakfast.
- Add a beet supplement to your cleanse, such as LifeSpa's "Beet Cleanse" formula.
- Take a teaspoon of chia seeds soaked in water for at least 5 minutes.
- Add 1 - 2 tablespoons of ghee to kitchari (especially if you have vata tendencies).

Loose Bowels
It is common to get some loose stools during the cleanse. This may be from the extra beets in your diet, the ghee or a fast-moving detoxification of the liver as more bile is released. Make sure you are drinking plenty of fluids. If it doesn't bother you and your energy level is fine, it will most likely pass. If if feels too excessive, try slowing down the ghee intake and discontinuing herbs that encourage elimination or bile production, such as beet or liver formulas.

Menstruation
It is best to time your cleanse when you are not menstruating. This is because menses will increase the vata quality already inherent to the cleanse. Each part of a woman's reproductive cycle has a different quality and dominant dosha associated with it. During the end of menses to ovulation kapha increases. From ovulation to menses pitta qualities increase. And, during the time of menses, vata is dominant. The cleanse itself temporarily increases vata due to the light, dry quality of the diet,

the herbs, and movement associated with the changes in physiology. Sometimes the increase of vata qualities will bring menses on sooner. Ideally, we are balancing the vata qualities by using oil in abhyanga massage, minimizing activities and using heat. However, if menses should happen during the cleanse, don't worry, you can adjust your cleanse using the balancing principles of Ayurveda.

First, stop taking any herbal supplements during your moon-time. Most cleansing herbs have a strong bitter quality, which increases vata. Second, decrease ghee intake. Menses itself has a detoxifying action on the body, and therefore having your moon-time during the purification phase may intensify the process. Taking less ghee will slow down the detoxification process. Third, be especially mindful to balance vata. This may mean adding more abhyanga massage, heat via steam saunas and baths, slowing down considerably, adding root veggies to kitchari and tending to your self with care and support.

Gallbladder Concerns

If you are dealing with gallbladder issues or have had your gallbladder removed, be sure to go slowly with the morning ghee during the Purification Phase. Listen to your body and notice how it responds. Also, using 4-5 capsules of triphala as a purgative rather than the castor oil will be your best choice.

Chapter 9
Rebuilding & Rejuvenation

"There are only two ways to live your life. One is as though nothing is a miracle. The other is as though everything is a miracle."

– Albert Einstein

Section 1: Rebuilding

<table>
<tr><td colspan="2">Rebuilding Phase - 3 Days (or more – until digestion feels strong again)</td></tr>
<tr>
<td>

Diet and Herbs:
- Follow the Digestive Reset protocol (below) using lemon, ginger and herbs.
- Continue following the simplified diet utilized during the Preparation Phase.
- Continue taking herbs and supplements for the cleanse until they are gone.
- Add probiotic foods and/or supplements to repopulate beneficial bacteria.
- Begin taking triphala: 1-2 capsules approx. 1 hour before bed and 1-2 capsules upon rising.
- Continue taking all medications.

</td>
<td>

Stress Management:
- Practice 10-15+ minutes of pranayama, yoga and/or meditation daily.

Self-Care:
- Spend the first day of this phase relaxing at home and keep food very simple, such as soups with whole grains and veggies.

</td>
</tr>
</table>

There are two main intentions of the Rebuilding Phase protocol:
1. Reignite digestive fire so you are able to digest and assimilate foods better.
2. Repopulate beneficial bacteria for improved immune system functioning and digestion.

FOOD FOR THE REBUILDING PHASE

Rebuilding Phase Protocol
- Go back to the Preparation Phase diet for at least 3 days: low fat, lots of veggies, and no gluten/dairy/sugar/red meat/alcohol or other hard to digest foods. Include plenty of fresh vegetables in your diet and have green smoothies and juices as much as possible. Continue eating the grated beet salad if you are enjoying it. You can gradually add some healthy fats, such as olive oil, coconut oil, flax oil, avocado oil and nuts to your diet at this time. Small amounts of lighter protein such as chicken can be added as well. Go slow with these heavier foods.
- **Digestive Reset:** Take a digestive boost about 10 minutes before each meal. Choose from the Ginger Lemon Appetizer (page 239) and/or 2 - 3 oz. of Lemon Digestive Tonic (recipe on page 150). For a stronger digestive boost, see enhancement option page 36.
- Introduce *small* amounts of probiotics into your diet. Good sources are probiotic supplements, sauerkraut or kim chi or other *live* fermented vegetable (start with taking just the brine and work your way up to the vegetable), miso, blue green algae, and tempeh. (Although we are staying clear of dairy in general, a small amount of kefir or lassi at the end of your midday meal can be introduced.)

STRESS MANAGEMENT & SELF-CARE FOR THE REJUVENATION PHASE

Continue to practice at least 10-15 minutes of yoga, stretching, meditation and/or prayer in the morning, or whenever it fits into your day. As you return to your maintenance diet and lifestyle, choose one or two self-care practices that you particularly enjoyed to integrate into your routine. Other self-care practices you can continue to focus on include:

- Maintain positive relationships
- Support digestion whenever needed using the Lemon Digestive Tonic and/or Ginger Lemon Appetizer
- Keep warm and out of wind (especially for vata types and during fall and early winter)
- Release perfection, judgment and criticism (especially for pitta types and during summer)
- Daily movement (in greater amounts for kapha types and during late winter and spring)

Rejuvenation Phase Checklist:
- ☐ Rejuvenating foods
- ☐ Slowly transition into a sustainable diet
- ☐ Optional herbs
- ☐ Stress Management - yoga, pranayama and meditation
- ☐ Self-care - as much as you can integrate

Sustainable Diet & Lifestyle

As we move into a regular diet, it is important to consider adjusting what we eat so that it is sustainable and balancing long-term. To do this, Ayurveda considers not just what to eat, but when and how, as well.

What
There are four main considerations in what to eat:

The first main consideration is that it is real food. This means that we try to eat home-cooked meals as much as possible, and that we stay away from packaged, processed, frozen foods. These foods tend to be lacking in life force (*prana*). Ayurveda has always been a strong advocate of eating prana-rich foods. These living foods provide a much more diverse and healthy microbiota. Numerous studies are now pointing to the primary importance of a diverse microbiota in digestive health, immunity and mental stability. Eating organic is important for this reason as well, as the diversity of helpful microorganisms is going to be higher with organic produce and animal products.

Second, we should eat foods that are in season. Looking at the season/constitution chart on page 132 will be helpful, as you can favor the foods that are listed for each season during that time. This overlaps with the "when" in Ayurveda, which recognizes the advantage to our beings when we eat in rhythm with the seasonal shifts. When we eat in season, we are eating the foods that we have evolved to metabolize over thousands of years. We see that each season provides the perfect balance to the dosha or quality that is prevalent in each season.

- **Spring**: Eating light, warming and detoxing foods in springtime will help to balance the sticky, heavy, moist qualities of kapha that are prevalent in spring. Think about what is naturally harvested during this time: we find early greens that are bitter and detoxifying, like dandelion, chicory, chard, and spinach. These are all very supportive foods for this time of year. We want to eat lots of warm spices to burn off excess kapha, such as ginger, hing, cumin, cinnamon, cardamom, turmeric, oregano, basil, black pepper. Additionally, eating more astringent types of foods, like legumes, helps pull excess mucous off of the intestinal walls.

- **Summer:** Eating primarily cooling, light foods in summer will balance the hot and oily qualities of pitta. Again, if we look at what is in season, there is an abundance of fresh fruit and vegetables. This should be the highest proportion of our diet. Protein should be light, such as chicken and fish that is caught in the summer months. Lighter grains like millet and rice are also good.

- **Fall and Early Winter:** To balance the cold, dry, and light qualities of vata, which are present in this season, we should focus on heavy, warm and moist foods. Traditionally, this is when humans eat meat, because it provides the fat necessary for keeping warm during the winter. Even if you are not a meat eater, you can take in more fat and protein with nuts, seeds and good oils. Eating root vegetables and heavier grains, like wheat and barley, are also balancing. Finally, eat warm food – in temperature and spiciness.

Third, we can consider our constitution and any imbalances present. When you know your constitutional tendencies, it is helpful to favor the foods in the chart on page 132 that correspond to balancing that dosha, even during other seasons. For example if you are vata, it is useful to keep dry, cold and light foods to a minimum while favoring moist, warm, and cooked foods. In the same way, when we experience an imbalance we can favor the foods that balance that dosha. This can sometimes be more complicated, as often more than one dosha is out of balance when we become sick. We highly recommend seeing an Ayurvedic practitioner to get an individualized diet and lifestyle plan for returning to wellness in this case.

Fourth, include all six tastes. According to Ayurveda, including all six tastes is the key to providing balanced nutrition to the body. The six tastes are: sweet, salty, sour, pungent (spicy), bitter and astringent (drying). Don't worry about getting all six tastes into every single meal, but if you have gotten all six tastes in a full day, you will feel more balanced and satiated. Our culture tends to favor sweet and salty food. Including all of the tastes in your diet leads to eating less and having a more balanced nutritious meal. A midday meal that satisfies you until dinner and leaves you fulfilled and energized will likely have all six tastes. The six tastes each stimulate different parts of digestion, and therefore create a fully operating metabolic machine. In addition, when you have all six tastes in your meal, you tend to feel more satiated and have less after-meal cravings. The following are some basic examples of the six tastes, but keep in mind that many foods have several tastes and qualities. These are just the prevalent ones.

- Sweet: sweet fruits, grains, meat, nuts and seeds, sweet veggies
- Sour: lemons and limes, yogurt, fermented foods
- Salty: salt, seaweed
- Pungent: peppers, onions, ginger, garlic, oregano, basil, cinnamon, cayenne
- Bitter: leafy green vegetables
- Astringent: legumes, pomegranate, apples, grape skins, cranberries

When

Just like all life forms on this planet, we have evolved around the circadian rhythms. And, we are intimately interconnected to the natural world. Therefore, along with the seasonal considerations, it is beneficial to follow daily rhythms in nature as well.

When the sun is the strongest during the day (between 10 am and 2 pm), our inner sun, or digestive fire, is strongest then, too. Therefore, it is best to have our biggest meal midday when our digestion can adequately break down and assimilate our food.

Oppositely, between 6 pm and 10 pm, when the sun is going down, our digestive strength is weak. Therefore, it is best to eat a light dinner as early as possible, so that we don't go to sleep with undigested food in our stomachs. In addition, it is important to wait at least three hours between meals. This allows us to use our digestive acids and enzymes efficiently before new food comes in. It is analogous to a clothing washing machine cycle: if you start putting in more dirty clothes before the washing cycle is complete, you end up with a bunch of clothing that hasn't been properly washed. Snacking is the equivalent to stacking more dirty clothes into the wash cycle. To facilitate the full cycle of digestion, food needs proper time through each digestive organ. Therefore, you want to eat a balanced, nourishing meal that leaves you satisfied until the next meal. If this is difficult, there may be a blood sugar imbalance. In this case, consult your practitioner or doctor.

How

This is probably the most important factor in eating well – honestly. When you

Rejuvenation Phase Recipes

Shopping List

The following is a shopping list with what you will need for all phases of your cleanse. This is not all-inclusive; please shop for the recipes you plan to make during your cleanse. Notice that the first section includes the "Essentials", and the second section includes "Optional" items. Once you have entered your cleanse into your calendar, we recommend spending a day planning and shopping for everything you will need. Look over the recipes, decide which ones you want to try and put the ingredients on your list. This will avoid the need to go out to the grocery store several times during your cleanse, allowing more time to rest and relax.

Essentials:
- Split mung beans (also called mung dal or moong dal)
- Whole grains:
    Basmati rice
    Quinoa
    Millet
    Buckwheat
    Amaranth
    Gluten-free oats
- Ghee (or unsalted organic butter to make your own)
- Beans and Legumes:
    Adzuki beans
    Black beans
    Garbanzo beans (chickpeas)
    Kidney beans
    Lentils (green, red, black)
    Navy beans
    Pinto beans
    Split peas
    White beans
- Lemons and Limes
- Fresh parsley, cilantro and/or basil
- Fresh ginger root

- Avocados
- Beets (a couple of bunches, with greens still on)
- Apples (several)
- Green vegetables, choose in-season when you can:
    Asparagus
    Broccoli
    Cabbage
    Celery
    Green beans
    Leafy veggies (spinach, chard, kale)
    Salad greens
    Zucchini
- Other vegetables, choose in-season when you can:
    Beets
    Carrots
    Cauliflower
    Cucumber
    Fennel bulb
    Garlic
    Onions
    Potatoes
    Peas, snap/shelling

- Radishes
  - Sea vegetables
  - Winter squash
  - Yams/sweet Potatoes
- Seeds:
  - Hemp
  - Sesame
  - Chia
  - Flax
  - Pumpkin
  - Sunflower
- Spices:
  - Asafoetida (hing or hingwastak)
  - Basil
  - Cardamom
  - Cinnamon sticks
  - Cloves, whole
  - Coriander seeds
  - Ground coriander
  - Cumin seeds/ground cumin
  - Fennel seeds
  - Fenugreek seeds
  - Mustard seeds
  - Oregano
  - Rosemary
  - Saffron
  - Sea salt (any high mineral type)
  - Thyme
  - Turmeric - ground/fresh
- Aloe gel or juice (for Liver Flush)

- Milk thistle seeds (for Liver Flush)
- Olive oil (for Liver Flush)
- Castor oil (hexane-free)
- Sesame oil or other oil for self-massage (and optional basti) - see pages 81 - 82 for recommendations on massage oils

Optional:
- Rice crackers or rice cakes - check labels and avoid preservatives, sweeteners or processed ingredients
- Fish (salmon, sardines in water, rainbow trout, etc.)
- Lean chicken or turkey (skinless, organic & free range)
- Unsweetened almond, rice, hemp or hazel-nut milk (small amount for ghee chaser)
- Fruit and berries
- Stone ground or Dijon mustard (check label, be sure there are no sweeteners, preservatives, colors , etc. – vinegar is okay)
- Bragg's or coconut aminos
- Vegetable stock without sweeteners or fats (Pacific brand or similar)
- Digestive teas, such as chai (green or herbal, using digestive spices like cardamom, cloves, etc.)
- Tulsi (holy basil) tea
- Epsom salts (for baths)
- Enema bag

What to Eat?

The recipes on the following pages are some of our favorites for all phases of the cleanse. They are separated into sections for the Preparation and Rebuilding Phases, the Purification Phase and, finally, the Rejuvenation Phase. If you are short on time, it is always an option to eat something quick and simple using ingredients from the shopping list. Some ideas are too simple to include as a recipe, but are still great ways to eat well during your cleanse, such as:

- Baked yam or potato
- Boiled beets with salt and pepper
- Steamed veggies, such as asparagus or broccoli
- Mashed avocado (on or with just about anything)
- Baked salmon with sea salt and pepper
- A hard boiled egg
- A simple salad with one of the dressings in the Dressings, Sauces and Spreads section

Eating out during the Preparation and Rebuilding Phases can also be challenging, but not impossible. Many restaurants can provide simple steamed vegetables and plain rice on request. Sushi restaurants usually offer miso soup and some Mexican restaurants may be able to provide black beans made without oils or lard.

Cooking for a Family While Cleansing

As parents, we both know how challenging it can be to cook meals for the rest of your family while you are cleansing. A couple tips we can share to make this easier:

- Cook your mung and rice separate so the rest of your family can have rice and steamed veggies. Add a baked salmon filet and dinner's done!
- Don't try to be perfect. It's okay if you cut corners and give your kids something that is quick and easy. Your relaxation is worth it. Many of the ideas listed above are things everyone can have.
- Encourage others to try some of your cleansing meals. They might actually enjoy it!

Preparation and Rebuilding Phase Recipes

Beverages

Digestive Teas

Classic Seeds Tea

4 Tbsp whole coriander seeds
4 Tbsp whole fennel seeds
2 Tbsp whole cumin seeds
1 Tbsp whole cardamom pods

1. Combine ingredients in a jar or bag and stir to combine.
2. To brew tea, place 1 Tbsp in a tea strainer, tea bag or thermos, add 12-20 oz. hot water and steep 20 minutes or more. Sip throughout the day.

Basic Ginger Tea

1 inch hunk of fresh ginger, sliced

1. Place ginger in the bottom of a mug or thermos.
2. Boil 12-20 oz. of water and pour over ginger. Cover and steep 20 minutes or more. Sip throughout the day.

Warming Digestive Tea

1 inch hunk of fresh ginger, sliced
½ tsp tulsi (holy basil) leaves
3–5 whole cardamom pods

1. Place all ingredients in a small pot and add 12-20 oz. water.
2. Simmer 7 minutes.
3. Strain and enjoy.

Liver Flush Smoothie

Take this once during the Preparation Phase.

2 Tbsp olive oil

2 Tbsp aloe gel or 1 cup aloe juice

1 lime or lemon, juiced

½ – 1 Tbsp milk thistle seed, ground (use a coffee grinder)

¼ tsp ground coriander

1. Combine all ingredients in a blender, blend and drink.

Wholesome Almond Milk

20 minutes, plus soaking time
Yields about 3 cups

1 cup raw almonds, soaked overnight, then drained

2 ¾ cups filtered water

1 date (optional), soaked and drained with ¼ cup soaking water reserved

1. Blanch almonds by covering them with boiling water, draining, and slipping off the skins.
2. Blend water, almonds and date/reserved water (if using) in a food processor on high until very smooth.
3. Strain through a cheesecloth. Squeeze to release all of the milk.
4. Store milk in an airtight container in the fridge for up to four days. Save pulp for baked goods (use similarly to almond meal) or add to hot breakfast cereals.

Quick & Healthy Hemp Milk

5 minutes
Yields about 2 cups

½ cup hemp seeds

1 ½ cups filtered water

¼ tsp vanilla extract (optional)

1. Place all ingredients in the work bowl of a food processor.
2. Process until smooth. Use immediately or store leftovers in an air-tight jar in the fridge for up to 4 days.

Green Apple Cleansing Cocktail

5 minutes
Yields about ½ cup

Apples help get the lymph system moving and detoxify the intestinal wall, while parsley helps remove heavy metals and other toxins from the body.

½ cucumber, peeled

1 medium green apple, such as Granny Smith

1 large handful of spinach

1 large handful of parsley

1. Cut all ingredients to fit into your juicer.
2. Juice, stir, and drink.

Beet & Cucumber Energy Juice

1 cucumber, peeled

3 medium carrots, scrubbed, tops and ends chopped off

2 stalks celery, washed

1 beet, scrubbed

2 leaves kale or chard, or a handful of spinach

1 handful parsley, washed

1 -to- 2 inch ginger root, scrubbed

½ lemon, peeled

1. Cut all ingredients to fit into your juicer.
2. Juice, stir, and drink.

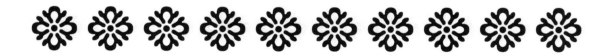

Savory All-Veggie Juice

5 minutes
Yields about ½ cup

3 large chard leaves with stalks

1 medium carrot, scrubbed, tops and ends chopped off

3 stalks celery, washed

Handful of spinach

1 handful parsley, washed

1 -to- 2 inch ginger root, scrubbed

¼ lemon, peeled

1. Cut all ingredients to fit into your juicer.
2. Juice, stir, and drink.

Lemon Digestive Tonic

5 minutes
Yields about 1 ¼ cups

½ cup lemon juice (about 2 large lemons)

¾ cup filtered water

1 Tbsp grated fresh ginger

Large pinch of sea salt

1. Combine all ingredients in a jar with a lid. Store in the refrigerator and drink 2 - 3 oz. 10 - 15 minutes before meals.

Elimination Tea

20 minutes, plus soaking time
Yields 1 quart

1 Tbsp slippery elm (cut and sifted)

1 Tbsp marshmallow root (cut and sifted)

1 Tbsp licorice root (cut and sifted)

1. Combine herbs and 2 quarts of water in a large jar or bowl and soak overnight, or about 6 - 12 hours.
2. Place everything in a pot and boil down until only a quart remains.
3. Strain and sip throughout the day to support movement of the bowels, alternating with plain warm water.

Digestive Lassi

¼ cup plain yogurt (homemade is best)

¼ tsp grated ginger

⅛ tsp ground cumin

⅛ tsp ground cardamom

Pinch sea salt

1 cup filtered water

1. Combine all ingredients in a glass and stir well. Enjoy after lunch during the Rebuilding Phase.

Golden Milk

5 minutes
Yields about 1 cup

1 cup almond milk

⅛ tsp nutmeg

¼ tsp turmeric

2 – 4 saffron strands

½ tsp raw honey (optional)

1. Combine everything except the saffron and honey in a small pot and heat over medium until warmed.
2. Remove from heat and add saffron and honey. Stir and drink about 30 minutes before bedtime.

Variation:
During the Rejuvenation Phase or when not cleansing, try this using non-homogenized grass-fed cow's milk.

Pineapple Digestive Tonic

Pulp from ½ small pineapple

2 limes, thinly sliced

4" hunk of ginger, sliced

1 tsp coriander seeds

1 tsp fennel seeds

6 cups filtered water

1. Combine all ingredients except for pineapple pulp in a large saucepan and bring to a boil. Lower heat and simmer about 15 minutes. Strain and return to pot.
2. Meanwhile, blend the pineapple pulp in a food processor. Add to pot and simmer an additional 5 minutes.
3. Serve warm or at room temperature.

Preparation and Rebuilding Phase Recipes

Breakfasts

Hot Quinoa Porridge

25 minutes
Yields about 2 ½ cups

1 cup quinoa, rinsed and soaked overnight, then drained

1 ½ cups water

Pinch of sea salt

½ cup chopped apples (optional)

Handful soaked raisins (optional)

Shredded coconut and/or seeds for garnish (optional)

½ cup unsweetened rice or almond milk

½ tsp cinnamon

1. Place quinoa, water and salt in a saucepan over high heat and bring to a boil.
2. Reduce heat, add fruit and/or raisins, if desired, and simmer until all the water is absorbed, about 20 minutes.
3. Place cooked quinoa into bowls, top with rice or almond milk, cinnamon and/or coconut. Serve hot.

Variations:
For a much faster version, try quinoa "flakes" or rolled quinoa, which cooks in 90 seconds.

For a savory version, cook in broth with a little salt and omit fruit and cinnamon. Serve with steamed veggies. When not cleansing, add some ghee, butter, or coconut oil just before serving.

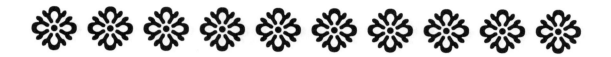

Sunny Steamed Eggs on Greens

10 minutes
Yields 1 serving

2 handfuls of chopped greens, such as kale, chard or cabbage

1 large organic egg

Sea salt and freshly ground black pepper, to taste

1. Heat a skillet over medium heat. Add greens and a splash of water and cover.
2. Cook about 2 minutes (longer for cabbage) then uncover, stir and create a nest in the center of the greens and crack egg into it. Add sea salt, black pepper and another splash of water (if needed), then replace lid.
3. Cook another 5-8 minutes, or until the yolk is cooked to desired firmness, adding more water as needed to keep greens from sticking to the bottom of the pan. Enjoy hot.

Blueberry Amaranth Porridge

30 minutes
Yields about 2 cups

2 cups water

Pinch of salt

⅔ cup amaranth (preferably soaked overnight)

½ tsp cinnamon

Unsweetened rice, almond, or hemp milk

1 Tbsp ground flaxseed

2 Tbsp chia seeds

½ cup blueberries, fresh or frozen

1. Bring water, salt and amaranth to a boil over high heat. Lower heat and simmer, stirring often to prevent sticking.
2. Cook 20-25 minutes until almost all the water is absorbed.
3. Add blueberries to the pot and cook another 5 minutes. Add cinnamon, milk and seeds right before serving. Enjoy hot.

Variation:
When not cleansing, add ghee, butter, or coconut oil before serving.

Morning Miso

1 cup water

1 small carrot, chopped small

1 stalk celery, chopped small

A few slices sweet onion

1 Tbsp wakame, soaked in warm water for 5 minutes

2 Tbsp miso paste, or to taste

Finely chopped chives or scallions

1. Place water, carrot, celery and onion in a medium pot and bring to a boil over medium heat.
2. Lower heat and simmer 5 minutes, or just until veggies are tender.
3. Turn off heat and allow to cool.
4. Add miso paste and wakame. Top with chives or scallions, if desired. Enjoy warm.

Breakfast Potatoes

25 minutes
Yields about 4 servings

½ cup water

4 large red skinned potatoes, cubed

1 large garnet yam, cubed

1 medium onion, sliced

3 cloves garlic, peeled and chopped

4 kale or collard leaves, torn

1 tsp sea salt, or to taste

1 tsp each dried basil, thyme and oregano

1 tsp smoked paprika

1. Place all ingredients except kale or collard leaves in a large skillet over medium heat.
2. Cook, covered, about 10 minutes, stirring often.
3. Add kale or collard leaves and cook another 10 minutes, or until fork-tender. Taste and adjust seasoning. Enjoy hot.

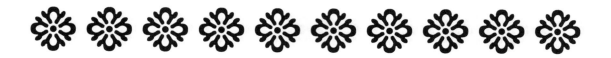

Creamy Hot Rice Cereal

15 minutes
Yields about 2 servings

2 cups water

Pinch of sea salt

½ apple, chopped small

½ cup brown rice farina (such as Bob's Red Mill)

½ tsp cinnamon

2 Tbsp chia seeds

Unsweetened rice, almond, or hemp milk (optional)

1. Bring water, salt and chopped apple to a boil over medium high heat. Add farina and cinnamon and reduce heat to low.
2. Cook approximately 8 minutes, stirring occasionally to keep cereal from sticking to the bottom of the pot.
3. Add chia seeds, stir well, and cook another 2 minutes, until seeds are soft, adding more water if necessary.
4. Divide into bowls and add milk, if using.

Variation:
Try this as a savory cereal by omitting apple and cinnamon and increase salt a bit.
When not cleansing, add ghee, butter, or coconut oil just before serving.

Chia Cereal

5 minutes
Yields 1 serving

3 Tbsp chia seeds

6 oz warm water or unsweetened almond, hemp, or rice milk

1 Tbsp hemp seeds

1 Tbsp tahini (sesame seed butter)

1 tsp pure vanilla extract

1 tsp cinnamon

Cooked apples and/or berries

1. Soak chia seeds in warm water or milk for 5 minutes.
2. Add remaining ingredients and enjoy.

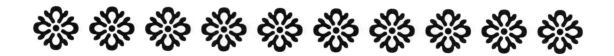

Cinnamon Apples & Raisins

25 minutes
Yields about 2 servings

According to Ayurveda, cooked apples for breakfast help create *ojas*, the final and most refined by-product of digestion, which contributes to enhanced vitality, strength and immunity. Fruits are best eaten on their own or before other breakfast foods.

2 medium sized organic apples, peeled and chopped

2 Tbsp organic raisins

¼ cup water

½ tsp cinnamon, or to taste

1 clove

1. Place all ingredients in a saucepan and bring to a boil.
2. Turn heat to low and cook covered until soft, about 20 minutes. Serve warm.

Variation:
When not cleansing, add 2 tsp ghee before serving.

Soaked Oat & Seed Cereal

25 – 35 minutes
Yields 6 cups cereal mix

4 cups organic quick oats

1 cup oat bran

¼ cup dried fruit (such as chopped dates or raisins)

1 cup ground seeds (any combination of sunflower, sesame, hemp, chia, flax)

1 Tbsp ground milk thistle (optional)

1 tsp cinnamon

½ tsp cardamom

¼ cup coconut flakes

To Prepare:
1 cup almond, rice, hemp or coconut milk

1. Place all ingredients except liquid in a bowl and stir until combined. (This mixture can be stored in an airtight container in the refrigerator until ready to use.)
2. To serve: Combine ½ cup cereal mix with 1 cup milk. Soak for at least 20 minutes. Enjoy immediately at room temp or cook gently over medium-low heat for 10 minutes.

Preparation and Rebuilding Phase Recipes

Veggies

Beet Liver Cleanser

10 minutes
Yields about 2 cups

2 raw beets, grated

Juice of 1 lemon

1 tsp lemon rind

1 tsp grated fresh ginger

1 small apple with peel on, grated

1 tsp mustard

Handful of fresh cilantro, chopped, for garnish (optional)

1. Combine all ingredients and stir well. Enjoy a little at each meal, ideally eating at least one beet per day during Preparation and Rebuilding Phases. Store remaining salad in an airtight container in the refrigerator.

Variation:
For a simpler version, just add lemon juice to beets and stir.

Seaweed Edamame Slaw

15 minutes
Yields about 4 servings

2 cups frozen shelled edamame

Sea salt

½ cup wakame

*2 cups thinly shredded green cabbage
(omit for vata)*

*½ large cucumber, seeded, cut into half
moons (omit for kapha)*

Juice of 2 large lemons

1 tsp sea salt

2 Tbsp toasted sesame seeds

1. Bring 4 cups of water to a boil over
   high heat. Add edamame and boil for
   4 - 5 minutes or until tender. Drain and
   sprinkle with sea salt. Set aside.
2. Meanwhile, soak wakame in warm water.
3. Toss cabbage, cucumber, lemon juice and
   salt together in a medium-sized bowl.
4. Add the edamame and seaweed, sprinkle
   with sesame seeds and toss. Taste and
   adjust seasoning.
5. Serve immediately or store in an airtight
   container in the fridge.

Variation:
When not cleansing, add 2 Tbsp toasted
sesame oil and 2 Tbsp rice vinegar, reduce
lemon juice by half.

Kneaded Kale & Avocado Salad

1 bunch kale, rinsed

½ tsp sea salt

¼ cup pumpkin or sunflower seeds, lightly toasted

1 avocado, diced

¼ cup red onion, finely sliced (optional)

Juice of ½ lemon

1. Stack rinsed kale leaves flat on top of each other and lay lengthwise in front of you. Starting with the edge closet to you, roll stack into a tight bundle. Slice into thin strips. (This is called *chiffonade*.)
2. Place kale and sea salt in a medium sized bowl and, using your hands, knead for two minutes until juicy and bright green.
3. Add remaining ingredients and toss. Serve immediately or store in an airtight container in the refrigerator.

Variation:
When not cleansing, add 2 Tbsp olive oil and 1 Tbsp balsamic vinegar; omit lemon juice.

Baked Yams & Apples

*2 medium-sized yams, cut into 2"
cubes*

*2 medium-sized apples, cut into 2"
cubes*

1 tsp ground cinnamon

Splash of water

1. Preheat oven to 350°.
2. Place all ingredients in a glass baking dish and cover. Bake 30 minutes or until tender when pierced with a fork, stirring once or twice during cooking. Enjoy hot or at room temperature.

Variation:
When not cleansing, add ghee, butter or coconut oil before baking.

Roasted Root Veggies

60 minutes
Yields about 4 – 6 servings

½ cup water

1 fennel bulb, sliced

2 medium carrots, cut into ¼" thick slices

1 large sweet potato, cut into ½" cubes

1 small onion, sliced

4 large red potatoes, cut into ¼" slices

1 tsp thyme

1 tsp rosemary

1 tsp oregano

1 tsp sea salt, or to taste

1. Preheat oven to 400°.
2. Place water in the bottom of an 11"x14" baking dish. Add veggies and herbs.
3. Bake 20 minutes, covered. Stir and bake another 20 minutes uncovered, or until fork-tender. Serve with rice or quinoa.

Variation:
Use whatever veggies and herbs you have to make this dish. When not cleansing, toss in 2 - 4 Tbsp avocado or coconut oil before baking.

Coconut & Apple Beets

25 minutes
Yields about 6 servings

½ tsp cumin seeds

¼ tsp mustard seeds

½ tsp coriander seeds

½ large leek, sliced

6 medium beets, cut into 1" cubes

2 apples, chopped

Handful beet greens, roughly chopped

1 inch hunk of fresh ginger, grated

½ tsp turmeric

2 Tbsp shredded coconut

Sea salt and freshly ground black pepper, to taste

1. In a dry skillet over medium heat, cook mustard, cumin and coriander seeds until they begin to pop.
2. Add leek, apples, beets, beet greens, ginger and turmeric. Add ¼ cup boiled water, lower heat and cover. Simmer until beets and apples are soft, adding more water as needed to keep from sticking to the bottom of the skillet.
3. Remove lid and add coconut, salt and pepper to taste. Serve warm or at room temperature.

Variation:
When not cleansing, cook seeds in ghee, butter or coconut oil until they pop, then follow the remainder of the recipe.

Spinach O-Hitashi

8 cups baby spinach, washed and stems removed

¼ tsp sea salt

Water to cover

2 Tbsp Bragg's or coconut aminos

1 Tbsp toasted sesame seeds

1. Fill a large pot with water, add salt and bring to a boil.
2. Add spinach and cook 20 seconds.
3. Drain into a colander and rinse with cold water to stop cooking process. Squeeze out excess water with your hands.
4. Divide spinach into 6 parts and roll into balls. Place on plates or a serving platter and drizzle a little liquid aminos over top each one.
5. Top with toasted sesame seeds and enjoy immediately.

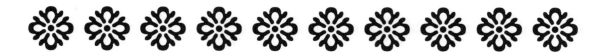

Gobo & Greens

2 large gobo root (also known as burdock), about 10" long, sliced into ⅛" thick coins

⅛ cup water

1 bunch of greens, any variety (kale, collards, chard, spinach, etc.), chopped

2 Tbsp tahini

Juice of ½ lemon

Sea salt to taste

1. In a skillet over medium heat, cook gobo root in water, covered, until almost tender, about 5-7 minutes, stirring occasionally. Add water as needed to keep from sticking to pan.
2. Meanwhile, in a small bowl, combine tahini, lemon juice and sea salt. Add just enough water to make a pourable dressing. Set aside.
3. When gobo is just about tender, add greens and cook another 4-5 minutes, until greens are soft and bright in color.
4. Add tahini sauce, stirring to coat. Serve immediately.

Variation:
When not cleansing, sauté gobo in olive or sesame oil for 5 minutes, add greens, cover and cook another 5 minutes. Add 1 Tbsp toasted sesame oil to dressing.

Mashed Cauliflower Potatoes

25 minutes
Yields about 6 servings

6 large red skin potatoes, cubed

1 large head cauliflower, chopped small

Water to cover

2 cloves garlic, minced (optional)

Sea salt and freshly ground black pepper, to taste

1. In a large pot, combine cauliflower and potatoes and boil in salted water until tender, about 15-20 minutes.
2. Drain most of liquid off and add garlic, if using. Blend using an immersion blender or an electric mixer. You can also use a hand masher for a chunkier texture or add more water to make the mixture smooth.
3. Add sea salt and pepper to taste. Serve hot.

Variation:
When not cleansing, add ghee, organic butter or good oil while mashing. The potatoes for this recipe can be peeled, if desired, but it is not necessary.

Edamame Lime Salad

10 minutes
Yields about 6 servings

3 cups shelled edamame

3 cups water

1 red bell pepper, diced

Juice of 1 lime

¼ tsp ground cumin

1 tsp sea salt, or to taste

¼ tsp smoked paprika

¼ cup fresh cilantro

¼ cup toasted sesame seeds

1. Place water in a medium pot and bring to a boil. Add edamame and cook 4-5 minutes, or until just tender. Drain and transfer to a mixing bowl.
2. Add remaining ingredients and toss to coat. Serve at room temperature.

Variation:
When not cleansing, add 2 Tbsp toasted sesame oil before tossing.

Vibrant Veggie Nori Rolls

15 minutes
Yields 4 rolls

4 red bell pepper slices, cut very thin

4 yellow bell pepper slices, cut very thin

Handful of mixed greens & herbs, such as arugula, borage, dill, parsley, cilantro, etc.

1 small carrot, shredded

1 medium avocado, cut into thin slices

Live sauerkraut

4 tsp toasted sesame seeds

4 sheets of nori

1. Lay nori sheets out flat on a dry surface with one of the corners pointing at you.
2. Place desired veggies in center of nori. Roll into a cone shape, from right to left, making sure the veggies don't fall out.
3. Wet the end of the nori with a little water and stick it to itself. Enjoy immediately. Serve along or with Creamy Oil Free Dressing (page 177) or Green Tahini Dressing (page 179).

Variation:
When not cleansing or during the Rejuvenation Phase, use some Probiotic Almond Cheese Spread (page 240) in these wonderful rolls.

Preparation and Rebuilding Phase Recipes

Dressings, Sauces & Spreads

Creamy Oil-Free Dressing

5 minutes
Yields about 1 ½ cups

1 cup unsweetened rice, soy or almond milk

¼ cup raw sunflower or pumpkin seeds

¼ cup fresh lemon juice (about 1 lemon)

1 Tbsp chia seeds

1 tsp Bragg's or coconut aminos

1 tsp Dijon or stone-ground mustard

3 Tbsp red or sweet onion, roughly chopped

3 Tbsp chopped fresh parsley

1. Place all ingredients in a blender and blend two minutes or until smooth. This dressing is best after a night in the refrigerator and will keep up to 5 days.

Honey Mustard Dressing

10 minutes
Yields about ¼ cup

¼ cup fresh lemon juice (about 1 lemon)

1 Tbsp Dijon mustard

1 Tbsp honey

1 clove garlic, finely grated or minced

1. Place all ingredients in a jar with a tight fitting lid. Shake well to combine.

Variation:
When not cleansing, add 3 Tbsp olive or flax oil.

Green Tahini Dressing

10 minutes
Yields about 1 cup

½ cup raw tahini

Juice of 1 lemon

Water to thin

1 clove garlic, grated or minced

Coconut aminos, Bragg's or sea salt, to taste

1 tsp ground cumin

3 Tbsp fresh parsley, finely minced

1. Combine tahini and lemon juice in a bowl or jar and stir until thick.
2. Add water slowly, a little at a time, until a pourable consistency is reached.
3. Add remaining ingredients and mix well, or add to a food processor to get the parsley very finely minced for a smoother (and more green) product.

Gourmet Guacamole

10 minutes
Yields about 4 servings

2 avocados, diced

2 medium tomatoes, diced

½ medium red onion, finely chopped

2 cloves garlic, grated or minced

Juice of 1 lemon or lime

½ tsp ground cumin

Sea salt to taste

½ cup fresh cilantro, chopped

1. Place avocado in a medium sized bowl and mash with a potato masher.
2. Add remaining ingredients and mix well. Serve immediately with rice crackers, polenta, beans or on top of a whole grain.

Variation:
To use as a dressing for green salads, thin with a little water, or use oil when not cleansing.

Cauliflower Curry Spread

15 minutes
Yields about 4 servings

1 cup chopped cauliflower

¼ cup water or unsweetened rice, soy or almond milk

1 clove garlic, minced

¼ tsp ground cumin

¼ tsp ground turmeric

⅛ tsp ground coriander

¼ tsp smoked paprika

⅛ cup red onion, finely chopped

¼ tsp sea salt

1. In a large pot with a steamer basket set inside, steam cauliflower until tender.
2. Place cauliflower and remaining ingredients in a food processor or blender and process until smooth. Serve warm or at room temperature.

Variation:
When not cleansing, add 2 - 3 Tbsp olive oil.

Homemade Lentil Dip

30 minutes
Yields about 2 cups

1 cup uncooked red lentils, soaked and rinsed

1 ½ cups water or veggie broth

¾ tsp sea salt

1 small onion, finely chopped

1 clove garlic, grated or minced

Juice of 1 lemon

½ tsp ground cumin

½ tsp smoked paprika

Handful of fresh cilantro or parsley, finely chopped

1. Bring water, salt and lentils to a boil in a medium sized pot. Lower heat and simmer uncovered, about 15 - 20 minutes or until very tender, adding more hot water if the lentils get too dry. When lentils are done, drain off any excess water. (A thick consistency is ideal.)
2. Add remaining ingredients and blend until smooth using a food processor or immersion blender, or mash by hand.

Variation:
When not cleansing, add a little olive oil before mashing.

Apple Chutney

2 organic apples, peeled, cored, and chopped

¼ cup raisins

½ tsp cinnamon

1" chunk of fresh ginger, grated

¼ tsp grated lemon rind

Juice of ¼ lemon

⅛ tsp salt

½ cup water

1. Place all ingredients in a medium sized pot and bring to a boil.
2. Lower heat and simmer, uncovered, for about 30 - 45 minutes, stirring occasionally, until very soft and a thick consistency is reached. You may need to add more water to keep from sticking to the bottom of the pot.

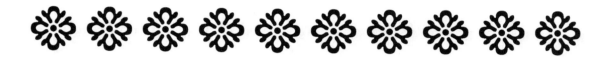

Pear Goji Chutney

35 minutes
Yields about 1 cup

2 organic pears, peeled, cored, and chopped

¼ cup goji berries

½ tsp cardamom

1" chunk of fresh ginger, grated

¼ tsp grated lime rind

Juice of ¼ lime

⅛ tsp salt

¼ cup water

1. Place all ingredients in a medium sized pot and bring to a boil.
2. Lower heat and simmer, uncovered, for about 30 - 45 minutes, stirring occasionally, until very soft, adding additional water as need to keep from sticking.

Cucumber Raita

1 cup organic whole yogurt

1 tsp ground fennel seeds

½ tsp ground cumin seeds

2 Tbsp fresh dill or cilantro

2 small cucumbers, peeled and diced

¼ tsp freshly ground pepper

½ tsp salt

1. In a skillet, dry roast fennel and cumin seeds over medium heat for 5 minutes. Grind coarsely using a mortar and pestle.
2. Add remaining ingredients and enjoy served with curried veggies or dal.

Variation:
For vata, add a ½ tsp ginger powder and ¼ tsp hing.

Gomasala Spiced Seed Mix

10 minutes
Yields about 1 cup

1 ½ Tbsp coriander seeds

1 ½ Tbsp fennel seeds

½ tsp cardamom seeds (green outer pods removed)

⅛ tsp black pepper (optional)

½ cup unhulled sesame seeds

1 ½ Tbsp sunflower seeds

½ tsp rock salt

½ cup hemp seeds

2 Tbsp coconut flakes

1 Tbsp maple sugar

1. Toast coriander, fennel, sunflower and sesame seeds in a heavy skillet on medium heat for about 5 minutes.
2. Add remaining ingredients and grind to desired texture in mortar and pestle. Store in an airtight container and enjoy after a meal or use as a seasoning on grains, veggies or dal.

Toasted Fennel Seeds

5 minutes
Yields ¼ cup

¼ cup fennel seeds

Pinch turmeric

Lemon juice

1. Heat a cast iron skillet over medium heat. Add fennel seeds and toast, stirring often, until their aroma is released.
2. Pour into a bowl and toss with enough lemon juice just to moisten and add turmeric. Allow to dry, then store in an airtight container. Enjoy a pinch of these after a meal as a refreshing digestive aid.

Mustard Tahini Dressing

2 Tbsp tahini

3 Tbsp miso paste

Juice of 1 ½ lemons

1 Tbsp stone ground mustard

3 Tbsp warm water

1. Combine all ingredients in a jar with a tight fitting lid. Stir or shake well until thoroughly mixed and a smooth texture is achieved. Use immediately or store in the refrigerator.

Parsley Sauce

5 minutes
Yields about ½ cup

½ cup packed fresh parsley

2 Tbsp lemon juice

2 garlic cloves

1 tsp fresh oregano (or ½ tsp dried)

¼ tsp sea salt

2 Tbsp water

1 inch peeled and sliced fresh ginger

1. Combine all ingredients in a food processor and blend until smooth.

Variation:
When not cleansing, reduce lemon juice to 1 Tbsp, add 2 tsp apple cider vinegar and replace water with 3 Tbsp olive oil.

Preparation and Rebuilding Phase Recipes

Soups

Blended Black Bean Soup

2 cups dry black beans, soaked 8 - 12 hours

1 tsp ground fennel

2 cups carrots or yams, washed and chopped small

2 cloves garlic, minced or grated

1 medium onion, chopped

1 tsp ground cumin

½ tsp each dried oregano, basil and paprika

1 tsp sea salt

Chopped parsley, cilantro and/or green onion for garnish.

1. Drain soaked beans, rinse, and fill pot with enough water to cover, plus one inch. Add ground fennel and cook until almost tender, about 1 ½ hours.
2. Add carrots or yams and all remaining ingredients and cook an additional 20 - 30 minutes until veggies are tender and beans are very soft.
3. Blend until smooth using an immersion blender or by transferring to a food processor, leaving some chunks if desired.
4. Return to heat and cook an additional 5 minutes. Serve garnished with chopped parsley, cilantro, and/or green onion.

Variation:
When not cleansing, sauté onion, carrot/yam and garlic in 2 Tbsp olive oil before adding to cooked beans.

Beautiful Borscht

1 hour
Yields about 4 servings

1 medium yellow onion, chopped

2 large carrots, chopped

2 stalks celery, chopped

2 large red skinned potatoes, cut into
1" - 2" cubes

4 medium beets, cut into 1" cubes

1 tsp each thyme, oregano and dill

1 ½ tsp sea salt

Freshly ground black pepper, to taste

4 cups water or broth

1 Tbsp lemon juice or balsamic
vinegar

1. Place all ingredients in a large pot and cook over high heat for 15 minutes.
2. Lower heat, cover, and cook for an additional 30 - 45 minutes, or until all vegetables are tender when pierced with a fork. Taste and adjust seasoning.
3. Serve hot or warm, garnished with chopped fresh parsley.

Variation:
Adding cooked rice or quinoa just before serving makes this a more hardy meal. When not cleansing, sauté onion, carrot and celery with thyme and oregano in 3 Tbsp olive oil before adding water, beets, potatoes and dill. Serve with a scoop of plain yogurt.

Creamy Fennel & Potato Soup

40 minutes
Yields about 2 – 4 servings

4 large potatoes, peeled and diced

1 medium onion, chopped

1 fennel bulb, chopped, plus fronds for garnish

2 cloves garlic, chopped

Salt to taste

1 ½ tsp dill weed

1. Place potatoes, onion, fennel, garlic and salt in a large pot and cover with water. Bring to a boil over high heat, then lower heat and simmer, approximately 20 minutes, or until potatoes are tender.
2. Drain off most of the cooking water (or less if you like a more brothy soup) and blend until smooth, using a food processor or immersion blender.
3. Add dill and stir to combine. Return to heat and cook for an additional 10 minutes. Taste and adjust seasoning if needed.
4. Pour into bowls, garnish with fennel fronds and serve hot.

Variation:
When not cleansing, sauté potatoes, onions, fennel and garlic in ghee, butter or olive oil before adding water to boil.

Curried Red Lentil Stew

40 minutes
Yields about 3-4 servings

1 ½ cups red lentils

3 cups water

1 tsp each cumin, turmeric, coriander, and sea salt

½ large onion, chopped

2 - 3 carrots, chopped

2 stalks celery, chopped

1 medium yam, chopped

4 cloves garlic, grated or minced

1 Tbsp grated fresh ginger

Juice of ½ lemon

Fresh cilantro, finely chopped, for garnish

1. Combine all ingredients except parsley in a large pot and bring to a boil over high heat.
2. Lower heat and cook, covered, for about 20 - 30 minutes or until lentils and vegetables are tender. Add lemon juice. Taste and adjust seasoning, if needed.
3. Ladle into bowls and garnish with cilantro. Serve hot.

Variation:
When not cleansing, sauté veggies and spices in 3 Tbsp ghee, butter or coconut oil, then add to cooked lentils and cook for another 10 minutes.

Quinoa Chili

45 minutes
Yields about 6 servings

2 cups cooked or canned beans

1 medium onion, chopped

2 stalks celery, chopped

1 medium carrot, chopped

1 cup sweet corn, fresh or frozen

4 large kale leaves, finely chopped

2 cloves garlic, minced or grated (optional)

1 tsp each oregano, cumin, and smoked paprika

Sea salt to taste

½ cup cooked quinoa

Fresh parsley or cilantro, finely chopped, for garnish

1. Place onion, celery, carrot, kale and oregano in a large pot and cover with water or broth. Bring to a boil and then lower heat and cook approximately 15 minutes.
2. Add corn, garlic, cumin, paprika, and salt and cook another 15 minutes.
3. Add beans and quinoa and cook another 10 - 15 minutes more, or until everything is heated through. Serve garnished with fresh cilantro or parsley.

Cauliflower Carrot Soup

35 minutes
Yields about 3 - 4 servings

1 medium head cauliflower, chopped

8 large carrots, chopped

Water or broth to cover

Sea salt to taste

1 Tbsp marjoram

1 Tbsp chopped fresh parsley, for garnish

1. Place cauliflower, carrots marjoram and salt in a large pot and cover with water or broth. Bring to a boil over high heat, then lower heat and simmer approximately 15 minutes, or until carrots are tender.
2. Drain off some of the liquid (more if you want a thicker, creamier soup and less if you want a thinner, brothy soup) then blend until smooth in a food processor or using an immersion blender.
3. Return to heat and cook another 15 minutes. Serve hot, garnished with fresh parsley, if desired.

Gingery Butternut Apple Soup

40 minutes
Yields 4 – 6 servings

1 medium Butternut squash, peeled, seeded, and cubed

4 medium sweet apples, peeled, cored and chopped

2 tsp ground ginger

1 tsp ground cardamom

2" chunk of fresh ginger, grated

Juice of 1 lime

Sea salt to taste

1. Place cubed squash and apples in a large stock pot and cover with water. Bring to a boil, lower heat and simmer until squash is tender, about 20 minutes.
2. Drain off most of water (more if you want a thick soup and less if you want a thinner, brothy soup) and blend until smooth using an immersion blender or food processor.
3. Add both gingers and cook another 15 minutes. Add lime juice just before serving. Enjoy hot.

Variation:
When not cleansing, add 1 can of coconut milk along with ginger.
For a savory version, omit apples and ginger and add onion and thyme. Replace lime juice with lemon juice and increase salt.

Immune Boosting Chicken Broth

8 hours, up to 2 days
Yields about 2 - 6 quarts

Homemade chicken broth is high in minerals, amino acids and other nutrients that support healthy bones, teeth and joints.

Carcass from a whole roasted chicken (or bones and sinew from several drumsticks)

1 small onion, roughly chopped

2 garlic gloves, smashed

2" hunk of ginger, roughly chopped

1 medium carrot, chopped

1 stalk celery, chopped

Fresh herbs, such as rosemary, thyme, sage or oregano (optional)

1 - 2 Tbsp sea salt

1. Place all ingredients except salt in a slow cooker or large stock pot and cover with water. Bring to a boil, then lower heat to simmer. (If using a slow cooker, set on low.) Cook 8 - 48 hours.
2. Add sea salt and stir to dissolve.
3. Strain liquid through a cheesecloth and discard solids.
4. Use broth immediately or store in canning jars in the refrigerator and reheat before using.

Super Immunity Veggie Broth

1 – 6 hours
Yields about 2 – 6 quarts

This recipe includes several ingredients that boost the immune system: shiitake mushrooms, onions, garlic, ginger and astragalus. If you're missing an ingredient or two, make this anyway! It will still be delicious and good for you.

½ onion, roughly chopped

2 cloves garlic, roughly chopped

2" hunk of ginger, roughly chopped

½ cup shiitake mushrooms (dried or frozen)

1 medium carrot, chopped

1 stalk celery, chopped

2 large kale leaves, chopped

1 Tbsp astragalus powder

Sea salt to taste

1. Place all ingredients except sea salt in a large stock pot on the stove or in a slow cooker and cover with water.
2. If using a stock pot, bring to a boil, then lower to simmer and cook 1 -2 hours. If using a slow cooker, cook on low for 2 – 6 hours. The longer it cooks, the more the flavors come through.
3. Add sea salt to hot broth and stir to dissolve.
4. Strain liquid through a cheesecloth and discard solids.
5. Use broth immediately or store in canning jars in the refrigerator and reheat before using.

Chicken Phở Broth

Phở (pronounced "fuh") is a traditional Vietnamese noodle soup typically made with beef or chicken bone broth. Because of the ingredients used, it is a wonderful digestive aid.

Carcass of a whole chicken (or several drumsticks – make sure it contains some bone and sinew)

1 medium onion, quartered

4" hunk of fresh ginger, halved length-wise and bruised

4–8 cloves garlic, peeled, whole

6 whole of each star anise, cloves and black peppercorns

1 Tbsp fennel seeds

1 - 2 Tbsp high mineral sea salt

1. Place all ingredients except salt in a large slow cooker. Cook on low for at least 8 or up to 48 hours.
2. Strain broth through a cheesecloth or fine sieve and return to slow cooker. Add sea salt and stir to dissolve. Taste and adjust seasoning.
3. Serve broth alone with a squeeze of lime juice or add steamed vegetables and fresh cilantro. This broth is also delicious over rice or quinoa.

Variation:
When not cleansing, add 4-6 Tbsp good quality fish sauce (without added sugar or preservatives, such as Red Boat brand) to the broth after straining and an hour before serving. Add thin rice noodles and chicken or tofu when serving soup. This broth can also be used to make Phở Quinoa Salad (page 212).

Spinach Avocado Soup

20 minutes
Yields 1 serving

2 stalks celery, washed and chopped

¼ cup sweet onion, chopped

¼ cup zucchini or green beans, chopped

2 kale leaves, chopped

½ cup water

½ cup baby spinach

1 medium avocado, diced

1 tsp sea salt, or to taste

½ tsp ground coriander

Freshly ground black pepper, to taste

1. Combine celery, onion, zucchini/green beans, kale, ground coriander and water in a medium pot. Bring to a boil, then lower heat and simmer about 5 minutes.
2. Add spinach and cook another 1-2 minutes.
3. Remove from heat. Add avocado and blend until smooth, using an immersion blender, food processor or blender. Add sea salt and black pepper. Taste and adjust seasoning. Serve warm or at room temperature.

Thick Split Pea Soup

1 cup dried split peas

6 cups water or broth

1 medium onion, chopped

2 medium carrots, chopped

2 cloves garlic, minced or grated

2 stalks celery, chopped

4 Tbsp fresh thyme (or 2 Tbsp dried)

2 fresh sage leaves (or 1 Tbsp dried)

Sea salt and freshly ground black pepper, to taste

Juice of ½ lemon, or to taste

Minced fresh parsley, for garnish (optional)

1 hour (more for slow cooker)
Yields about 6 servings

1. Combine peas, water, veggies, thyme and sage in a stock pot on the stove or in a slow cooker.
2. If using a stock pot, bring to a boil, then lower to simmer and cook about 45 minutes, or until peas are very soft, stirring occasionally. If using a slow cooker, cook on low for 8 hours.
3. Add lemon juice near end of cooking, along with sea salt and black pepper, and simmer another 10 minutes. Serve hot, garnished with parsley.

Variation:
When not cleansing, sauté vegetables in 2 Tbsp olive or avocado oil with herbs until beginning to soften, about 5-8 minutes. Add ½ cup water or broth and stir. Add split peas and remaining water or broth, bring to a boil, then lower heat to simmer and cook until peas are tender, stirring occasionally.

Creamy Asparagus Soup

40 minutes
Yields 2 - 4 servings

2 quarts water or stock

4 medium potatoes cut into 2" chunks

1 small head cauliflower, chopped

½ medium onion

2 cloves garlic, roughly chopped

2 bunches asparagus, chopped and ends trimmed off

2 stalks celery, chopped

½ tsp dried thyme

½ tsp dried dill

2 tsp sea salt, or to taste

Freshly ground black pepper, to taste

Juice of ½ to 1 lemon

1. Combine water or stock, potatoes, cauliflower, onion, garlic, celery, thyme and sea salt in a large pot. Bring to a boil over high heat. Lower heat to simmer, cover and cook 10 minutes, stirring occasionally.
2. Add chopped asparagus and cook another 10 minutes, or until tender.
3. Remove from heat and allow to cool slightly. Blend using an immersion blender or in batches using a food processor or blender.
4. Return to heat, add pepper, lemon and dill and cook another 10 minutes over medium-low heat.
5. Serve warm or at room-temperature, garnished with fresh herbs or arugula leaves.

French Lentil Dal

35 minutes, plus soaking time
Yields about 3 - 4 servings

1 cup French lentils

4 cups of water

3 cloves garlic, finely chopped

Pinch of hing or ¼ tsp hingwastak

1 tsp sea salt

1 tsp each turmeric, cumin, coriander and fenugreek

¼ tsp cayenne (omit for pitta)

1 Tbsp freshly grated ginger

2 - 4 collard leaves, chopped small

Handful of fresh basil

Juice of ½ lemon

1. Soak lentils in warm water for 2 - 6 hours, then rinse and drain.
2. Combine all ingredients except lemon juice, collard leaves and basil in a large pot and bring to a boil over medium high heat. Lower heat, cover and simmer about 1 hour, or until lentils are very soft. Alternatively, cook in a slow cooker on high for 3 hours.
3. In the last 15 minutes of cooking, add collard greens and basil.
4. Add the lemon juice and serve warm.

Variation:
When not cleansing, sauté garlic and spices in 2 Tbsp coconut oil for 3-5 minutes. Add lentils, coat with oil/spice mix and cook over low heat another 3-5 minutes. Add water and cook as instructed above. Add 1 can of coconut milk during the last 15 minutes of cooking.

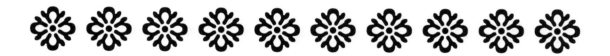

Preparation and Rebuilding Phase Recipes

Grains

Guide to Cooking Grains

Basic cooking instructions for whole grains:
1. Measure the grain, check for pebbles, bugs or other foreign material and rinse in cold water using a fine mesh strainer.
2. Soak grains 6 hours or overnight, if possible.* (Soaking white rice is not necessary.)
3. Drain, rinse and add grains to recommended amount of water and bring to a boil.
4. Reduce heat, cover and simmer for the suggested amount of time, without stirring during the cooking process. (Although rolled oats, amaranth and polenta should be stirred.)

1 cup of dry grain yields about 2 to 4 servings.

1 Cup Grains	Water	Approx. Cook Time
Brown rice	2 cups	40 - 50 minutes
White rice (basmati)	1 ½ cups	15 - 20 minutes
Buckwheat (kasha)	2 cups	20 - 30 minutes
Oats (whole groats)	3 cups	45 - 60 minutes
Oatmeal (rolled oats)	2 cups	15 - 20 minutes
Cornmeal (polenta)	3 cups	20 - 25 minutes
Millet	2 cups	25 - 35 minutes
Quinoa	2 cups	20 - 25 minutes
Amaranth	3 cups	25 - 30 minutes

Cooking times are approximate; length depends on how high the heat is. If you're unsure about cooking time, lift the lid and check the water level halfway through cooking, then again toward the end, making sure there is still enough water to keep the grains from sticking to the bottom of the pot.

---

* Most grains contain phytic acid in varying amounts, which can reduce the body's ability to absorb the calcium, iron, magnesium, and zinc in the grains. Therefore, many resources recommend soaking grains in water for at least 6 hours or overnight, to cut down on the amount of phytic acid they contain. Apple cider vinegar or lemon juice can be added to the soaking water (½ - 1 Tbsp) to further break down the phytic acid. Soaking grains will alter their texture - it makes short grain brown rice softer and easier to chew, but it may make amaranth or millet mushy. Many traditional cultures typically soak grains until they ferment to aid in digestibility.

Southwest Quinoa & Avocado Pilaf

10 minutes
Yields about 2 servings

1 cup cooked quinoa

¼ cup finely minced red onion

1 small red bell pepper, chopped small

½ cup sweet corn, fresh or frozen

1 avocado, diced

Juice of 1 lime

Sea salt, to taste

½ tsp ground cumin

½ tsp ground coriander

½ tsp smoked paprika

1. In a small pot over high heat, bring 2 cups of water to a boil. Add sweet corn, lower heat and cook until tender, about 4-5 minutes. Drain.
2. Combine all ingredients in a large bowl and stir to coat. Taste and adjust seasoning, as needed.

Variation:
For added protein, add 2 cups black beans. When not cleansing, add 2 Tbsp olive oil.

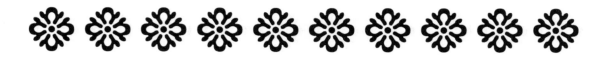

Quinoa Tabbouleh

15 minutes
Yields about 2 servings

1 cup cooked quinoa

1 medium tomato, diced

1 medium cucumber, quartered and diced

1 ¼ cups minced fresh parsley

½ cup minced fresh mint

Juice of 1 lemon

1 tsp ground cumin

Sea salt to taste

1 green onion, finely chopped

1. Combine all ingredients in a medium sized bowl and mix well. Serve at room temperature or chilled.

Variation:
When not cleansing, add 2 Tbsp olive oil before tossing.

Garlicky Millet Mash

30 minutes
Yields about 4 – 6 servings

1 cup millet, soaked and drained

1 cup chopped cauliflower

2 cloves garlic, chopped

3 cups water

Salt and pepper to taste

Fresh parsley, finely chopped

1. Place millet, cauliflower, garlic and water in a large pot and bring to a boil over high heat.
2. Lower heat and cook, covered, stirring occasionally until all water is absorbed and a mashed-potato-like consistency is reached, about 20 minutes.
3. Season with salt and pepper to taste and top with fresh parsley. Serve hot.

Variation:
Try replacing the cauliflower with yam or sweet potato. You can also add thyme or oregano to the cooking water, or add ground cumin or paprika just before serving. This is a perfect recipe to get creative with! When not cleansing, serve topped with ghee, butter or olive oil.

Millet Polenta

1 ½ hours
Yields one 9" x 11" baking dish

5 cups water

1 cup millet

*1 cup coarse ground cornmeal
(polenta)*

2 tsp sea salt

1. Lightly oil a large baking dish. Place water and millet in a large pot and bring to a boil. Lower heat to medium, stir in polenta and cook for 20 - 30 minutes, stirring often with a wooden spoon, until a very thick, smooth consistency is reached. Add sea salt and stir to combine.
2. Pour cooked polenta into prepared baking dish and let set for 1 hour in the refrigerator, or until firm and holds together when cut.
3. Cut into squares or triangles and serve alone or topped with beans, soft cooked vegetables, or a thick stew. This has infinite possibilities.

Variation:
Try adding herbs to the cooking water, like rosemary, thyme, oregano, or basil, or add ground spices before pouring into the baking dish, like cumin, coriander, or paprika. Also try this with chopped kalamata olives mixed in. When not cleansing, add 4-6 Tbsp organic butter or olive oil to the mixture just before transferring into prepared dish.

Zesty Beet & Quinoa Pilaf

45 minutes
Yields about 6 servings

3-4 medium beets, quartered

2 cups cooked quinoa

½ cup toasted pumpkin seeds

½ cup red onion, thinly sliced

2 tsp Dijon mustard

Juice and rind of 1 large lemon

2 Tbsp water

2 cloves garlic, minced or grated

½ tsp each ground cinnamon, cumin & coriander

½ cup chopped cilantro

Sea salt and freshly ground black pepper, to taste

1. Place beets in a large pot and cover with water. Bring to a boil, lower heat and cook until tender when pierced with a fork, about 20 - 30 minutes. Drain water, let cool and slip off skins. Cut into ½" thick triangles.
2. While beets are cooking, prepare the dressing: Combine mustard, lemon juice & rind, water, garlic and ground spices in a jar with a tight-fitting lid and shake well.
3. In a large bowl, combine quinoa, beets, red onion, and seeds. Pour dressing over top and toss to coat.
4. 4. Mix in cilantro, salt and pepper. Serve warm or chilled.

Variation:
When not cleansing, add 4 Tbsp olive oil to the dressing and omit water. Also try this using walnuts or pecans during fall and winter.

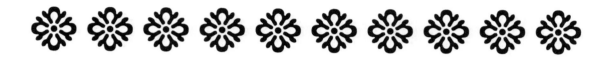

Phở Quinoa Salad

1 cup uncooked quinoa, soaked and drained

2 cups phở broth (page 200)

½ cup thinly shredded cabbage (omit for Vata)

½ cup chopped scallion

½ cup chopped fresh basil

½ cup chopped cilantro

1 small carrot, grated

Juice of 2 limes

2 Tbsp Bragg's or coconut aminos, or to taste

1. Combine quinoa and broth in a large pot. Bring to a boil, then lower heat and cook until all the water is absorbed, about 25 minutes.
2. Combine remaining ingredients in a large serving bowl and toss to coat. Serve warm or at room temperature.

Variation:
When not cleansing, add 3 Tbsp toasted sesame oil before tossing.

Whole Grain Nori Rice Balls

40 minutes, plus soaking time
Yields about 15 balls

¾ cup short grain brown rice

⅛ cup millet

⅛ cup amaranth

⅛ cup toasted sesame seeds

1 ½ cups filtered water

Nori sheets, cut into long, thin strips

Bragg's or coconut aminos for dipping (optional)

1. Soak grains 6-12 hours. Drain.
2. Place grains in a medium pot and add water. Bring to a boil, then lower heat and simmer until all water is absorbed, about 25 minutes, stirring occasionally to keep from sticking to pot. Allow to cool.
3. When grains are cool enough to handle, roll into balls, roll in sesame seeds, then wrap with a strip of nori. Fasten nori by wetting the end with a little water, then sticking it to itself around the ball.
4. Serve with Bragg's or coconut aminos for dipping.

Citrus Rice Summer Salad

2 cups cooked brown rice

½ medium bell pepper, diced

*½ cup red cabbage, thinly shredded
(for vata, omit or use chard or
spinach)*

*½ cup chopped fresh cilantro and/or
basil*

½ cup chopped green onion

Juice of 1 – 2 lemons or limes

Sea salt to taste

½ tsp ground cumin

*½ cup toasted pumpkin seeds
(optional)*

1. Place all ingredients in a large mixing bowl and toss to coat.

Variation:
When not cleansing, add 2 Tbsp olive or avocado oil before tossing.

Preparation and Rebuilding Phase Recipes

Main Dishes

Black Beans with Avocado & Corn

10 minutes
Yields about 1 cup

1 cup cooked or canned black beans

1 avocado, diced

½ cup corn, fresh or frozen

Juice of 1 lime

½ tsp each cumin and smoked paprika

¼ cup minced fresh cilantro

1. In a medium pot, bring 2 cups water to a boil. Add corn and cook about 4-5 minutes, or until tender. Drain.
2. Combine all ingredients in a medium sized bowl and mix well.

Variation:
When not cleansing, add 1 - 2 Tbsp olive or avocado oil before mixing.

Southwest Squash

45 minutes
Yields about 4 servings

4 cups peeled, seeded and chopped winter squash - Butternut, Hubbard, Kuri, or similar

1 medium yellow onion, chopped

1 tsp oregano

1 ½ cups cooked or canned black beans

½ cup grated zucchini

½ cup kale, finely chopped

2 cloves garlic, grated or minced

½ tsp each cumin and chili powder

Juice of 1 lime

Salt and pepper to taste

¼ cup finely chopped cilantro

1. Place squash, onion and oregano in a large pot with enough water to cover and bring to a boil over high heat.
2. Lower heat and cook until squash is just tender, about 20 minutes. Drain.
3. Meanwhile, in a separate pot combine beans, zucchini, kale, garlic, spices, salt, and lime juice and warm over medium heat. Add enough water to keep from sticking to pot. Add cooked squash and stir well.
4. Allow to cook another 15 minutes, until all the flavors have mingled. Serve warm, topped with cilantro. This is wonderful served with rice, quinoa or polenta.

Baked Rosemary Chicken & Potatoes

45 minutes
Yields about 4 servings

4 skinless, boneless chicken breasts or thighs, cut into large pieces

3 cloves garlic, chopped

1 onion, sliced

2 – 4 medium potatoes, cut into 2" cubes

1 Tbsp fresh rosemary, finely minced (or 2 tsp dried rosemary)

1 – 2 lemon wedges

Sea salt and freshly ground black pepper, to taste

1 cup of water

1. Preheat oven to 425°. Rinse chicken and pat dry with paper towels. Place in a large baking dish.
2. Add garlic, onion and potatoes to baking dish and add water. Sprinkle with rosemary and top with a squeeze of lemon.
3. Bake, covered, approximately 20 minutes.
4. Remove cover, stir, rotate dish and bake another 20 minutes or until chicken is cooked all the way through. A meat thermometer stuck into the thickest part of the meat should read at least 165°. Serve hot with a side of green veggies.

Basil Chickpea Summer Salad

10 minutes
Yields about 2 servings

1 cup cooked or canned chickpeas

¼ cup fresh basil leaves, chopped

Juice of 1 lemon

⅛ cup red bell pepper, thinly sliced

1 tsp each ground cumin and coriander

Salt and pepper to taste

1. Combine all ingredients in a medium sized bowl and mix well. Marinate 30 minutes before serving.

Variation:
Try omitting lemon juice, cumin and coriander and serve this instead with Green Tahini Dressing (page 179).
When not cleansing, add 1 - 2 Tbsp olive or avocado oil before mixing.

White Bean & Tomato Medley

10 minutes
Yields about 2 servings

1 cup cooked or canned white beans

1 cup chopped fresh parsley

2 ripe tomatoes, chopped

Juice of ½ lemon

½ red onion, minced

¼ tsp sea salt, or to taste

1. Combine all ingredients in a medium sized bowl and mix well.

Variation:
Try omitting onion and lemon juice and toss with Creamy Oil Free Dressing (page 177) instead.
When not cleansing, add 1 - 2 Tbsp olive oil before mixing.

Sardines with Shaved Fennel

10 minutes
Yields about 2 servings

1 large fennel bulb

Juice of ½ lemon

¼ cup chopped fresh parsley or basil

Sea salt and pepper to taste

1 tin sardines in water

Handful toasted seeds

1. Slice fennel bulb very thin using a mandoline or a very sharp knife.
2. Combine all ingredients in a medium sized bowl and mix well. Marinate 30 minutes before serving.

Variation:
If you don't have a fennel bulb, try this with zucchini.

Collard-Wrapped Burritos

45 minutes
Yields about 3 - 6 servings

6 large collard leaves

2 cups cooked or canned beans (black, pinto, adzuki, navy, etc.)

½ tsp each ground cumin, chili powder, and smoked paprika

Sea salt to taste

2 cups of your favorite vegetables, chopped and steamed

Handful fresh salad mix

Chopped fresh cilantro

Minced green onion

1. Lightly steam collard leaves until they are flexible and can bend without breaking.
2. Meanwhile, warm beans in a medium sized pot and season with ground spices and salt.
3. Lay collard leaves out on the counter and place in each one: a scoop of beans, a scoop of cooked vegetables, a layer of salad mix and a sprinkle of fresh cilantro. Top with green onion.
4. Roll collard leaves up and place on plates, seam-side down. Serve immediately.

Quinoa Hummus Salad

2 cups cooked quinoa

1 ½ cups cooked or canned chickpeas

1 cup Green Tahini dressing (page 179)

Sea salt to taste

2 large carrots, grated

Handful chopped fresh parsley

1. Combine all ingredients in a large bowl and stir to coat. Serve warm, at room temperature or slightly chilled.

Ginger Lemon Salmon

20 minutes
Yields 4 servings

4 salmon fillets, fresh or frozen and thawed

½ lemon, sliced thin

2" hunk of fresh ginger, grated

1 Tbsp Bragg's or coconut aminos, or sea salt to taste

1. Preheat oven to 375°.
2. Prepare salmon by rinsing, patting dry and placing on an oiled baking sheet or dish.
3. Rub with aminos or salt, add ginger and then top with lemon slices.
4. Bake until salmon begins to flake, about 15 - 18 minutes, rotating once during cooking.

Miso Glazed Salmon

4 salmon fillets, fresh or frozen and thawed

2 Tbsp miso paste

Juice of ½ lemon

Warm water

1. Preheat oven to 375°.
2. Prepare salmon by rinsing, patting dry and placing on an oiled baking sheet or dish.
3. Bake about 15 minutes, rotating once during cooking.
4. Meanwhile, prepare the glaze: In a small bowl stir together miso paste, lemon juice and enough warm water to make a thick spreadable paste.
5. Remove salmon from oven and cover each fillet with a layer of miso glaze, about 2 tsp on each.
6. Turn broiler on high and move oven rack to the highest position, about 8" from the top. Return salmon to oven and broil for 3 - 4 minutes, until the top just begins to crisp. Remove from oven and serve.

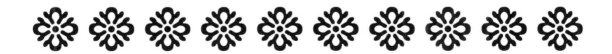

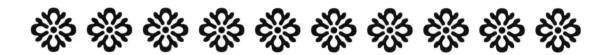

Baked Rainbow Trout with Fresh Herbs

20 minutes
Yields about 4 servings

4 small rainbow trout fillets (or 2 boned and butterflied trout)

Sea salt and freshly ground pepper

1 lemon, half sliced & half cut in wedges

Fresh tarragon, dill and/or rosemary, chopped

1. Preheat oven to 450°.
2. Salt and pepper both sides of fillets and lay each one on a large sheet of aluminum foil (large enough to wrap each entire fillet or fish).
3. Sprinkle with chopped fresh herbs and top with lemon slices.
4. Fold foil over each fillet and cinch the edges together. Place on a baking sheet and bake for 10-15 minutes, until the flesh is opaque and pulls apart when tested with a fork.
5. Serve with juices poured over top and extra lemon wedges.

Purification Phase Recipes

More Meal Ideas for the Purification Phase

Don't feel that you have to limit yourself during the Purification Phase to just the recipes in this section. As with the Preparation and Rebuilding Phases, you can always add steamed fresh vegetables to your meal, cook veggies into your kitchari or have a simple baked yam topped with shredded coconut. Particularly during the last few days of the Purification Phase, you might begin to feel like you can't possibly eat another bite of kitchari. That's fine - it doesn't mean you have to give up on your cleanse. Eat something else that is healthy and light.

Recipes from the Preparation and Rebuilding Phases that are also appropriate for the Purification Phase include:

For breakfast:
- Hot Quinoa Porridge
- Blueberry Amaranth Porridge
- Morning Miso
- Creamy Hot Rice Cereal
- Chia Cereal
- Cinnamon Apples & Raisins

To add variety:
- Beet Liver Cleanser
- Baked Yams & Apples
- Roasted Root Veggies
- Coconut & Apple Beets
- Spinach O-Hitashi
- Apple Chutney
- Pear Goji Chutney
- Toasted Fennel Seeds
- Beautiful Borscht

- Cauliflower Carrot Soup
- Gingery Butternut Apple Soup
- Immune Boosting Chicken Broth
- Veggie Broth
- Chicken Phở Broth
- Garlicky Millet Mash (omit garlic)
- Whole Grain Nori Rice Balls
- Southwest Squash (omit black beans)

For extra protein:
- Baked Rosemary Chicken (omit potatoes & onions)
- Ginger Lemon Salmon
- Miso Glazed Salmon
- Baked Rainbow Trout with Fresh Herbs

You can also try different combinations to make your kitchari something new each day.

Some ideas to liven up your kitchari include:

- Add veggies to the cooking pot - add harder vegetables like carrots when adding the mung and rice; soft vegetables like zucchini can be added during the last ten minutes of cooking. Some of our kitchari recipes call for veggies, some do not, but all of them can be cooked with veggies in them. You can alter the recipes by using veggies you like best. If a recipe calls for a veggie you don't have or don't enjoy, omit it or use something else.
- Add condiments to your kitchari. Condiments you can use while cleansing include grated fresh ginger, shredded coconut, fresh herbs (such as cilantro, basil or parsley), toasted seeds, and lemon or lime wedges.
- Try cooking the mung and rice separately - cook the rice according to the basic recipe on page 206 in the Grains section; cook the mung using a 1 cup mung to 2 ¾ cups water ratio.
- Add ghee to your kitchari. If you are dealing with a vata imbalance or have a vata-predominant constitution, adding ghee may be very helpful. (See page 101 - 102 and the constitution quiz in Chapter 2 for more information on this.) If at anytime you are feeling ungrounded or anxious (signs of vata imbalance), adding a little ghee to the dish will help balance that dosha.

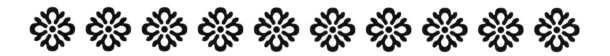

Ghee

20 – 40 minutes
Yields about 4 servings

1 pound unsalted or cultured organic butter

1. Place butter in a medium saucepan and slowly melt over medium heat.
2. Allow to boil, then reduce heat to very low and simmer uncovered and undisturbed for 20 - 30 minutes. The butter will foam and make crackling noises. The milk solids will slowly settle to the bottom and resemble fine toasted bread crumbs, leaving a pale golden liquid on top.
3. Once the milk solids have settled, immediately strain through a cheesecloth into a clean glass jar. This will stay fresh at room temperature for a few weeks, but you may refrigerate if you choose.

Classic Kitchari

¾ *cup basmati rice (brown or white, or substitute quinoa)*

¾ *cup yellow split mung beans (mung dal)*

1 tsp black or brown mustard seeds

1 tsp cumin seeds

2 pinches hing or asafoetida or hingwastak

½ tsp turmeric

¼ tsp ground coriander

½ inch stick of cinnamon (optional)

½ tsp sea salt

4 cups water

1. Wash rice and mung dal. Soak mung for an hour, if possible.
2. In a medium pot, dry roast mustard and cumin seeds, stirring until they begin to pop. Add remaining spices, salt, mung, and rice, and stir for a few minutes.
3. Add water and bring to a boil. Boil uncovered, stirring occasionally, about 5 minutes.
4. Turn heat down to low and cook until tender, about 20 - 30 minutes, stirring occasionally.

Variations:
When not cleansing, toast seeds in 4 Tbsp ghee, butter, or coconut oil before adding mung and reamining spices. Condiments when not cleansing can also include toasted and chopped nuts and pickled vegetables.

Pitta Pacifying Mung Dal

30 - 35 minutes
Yields about 3 - 4 servings

1 cup mung dal

3 cups water

1 tsp sea salt

½ tsp fennel seeds

½ tsp ground coriander

½ tsp basil

½ tsp turmeric

Pinch of hing or asafeotida

Lime wedges

Chopped fresh cilantro

Shredded coconut (unsweetened)

1. Place mung, water, sea salt and fennel seeds in a pot.
2. Bring to a boil over medium-high heat, lower heat to simmer and cook, stirring often, until almost all the water is absorbed, about 20 minutes.
3. Stir in remaining spices and cook another 5 minutes.
4. Squeeze lime juice into mung and stir well. Serve hot, garnished with cilantro and coconut.

Vata Comfort Kitchari

30 – 40 minutes
Yields about 3 – 4 servings

2 tsp ghee

1 Tbsp each coriander and cumin seeds

½ cup split mung beans

½ cup brown or white basmati rice

Pinch of hing

1 tsp sea salt

4 cups boiled water

1 tsp each cinnamon and cardamom

½ tsp dried ginger

¼ tsp cloves

1 inch fresh ginger, grated

1 inch fresh turmeric root, grated

½ sweet potato, cut into cubes

½ apple cut into pieces

½ cup peas, fresh or frozen

2 handfuls spinach

1. In a large pot, cook seeds in ghee over medium heat until they pop. Add mung beans, rice, hing and salt and stir for 5 minutes.
2. Add 4 cups boiled water and the rest of the spices. Simmer, covered, for 20 minutes, stirring occasionally.
3. Add apple and sweet potato, stir and cook for another 15 minutes.
4. Add the peas and spinach, stir and cook for 5 more minutes, until all the water is absorbed and everything is cooked through. Serve hot, garnished with lime juice, cilantro, and coconut flakes.

Variations:
Any constitution type can enjoy this recipe. For pitta and kapha types, omit ghee.

High Protein Kitchari

45 minutes
Yields about 3 - 4 servings

¾ cup split mung beans (soaked and rinsed)

¼ cup uncooked quinoa (soaked and rinsed)

½ tsp hing (asafeotida)

4 cups boiled water (if you want it more solid/less soupy, use 3 cups boiled water)

1 tsp ground turmeric

1 tsp ground cumin

1 tsp ground coriander

½ tsp fennel

½ tsp fenugreek

2 Tbsp curry leaves (optional)

1 tsp himalayan or sea salt

1 cup chicken broth

1 cup frozen or fresh peas

1. On medium low heat, add the drained quinoa and mung beans to a medium sized pot.
2. Stir in ½ the salt and the rest of the spices. Completely coat the bean-grain mixture with spices, stirring with a wooden spoon occasionally about 5 minutes. (If you are vata type or vata imbalanced, this would be the time to add ghee.)
3. Add the boiled water and bring to a simmer. Cover and cook for 30 minutes.
4. Add the chicken stock and salt to taste and simmer with lid partially on for another 5 minutes.
5. Add the peas and simmer 5 more minutes.
6. Garnish with Gomasala Spiced Seed Mix (page 186) and fresh chopped ginger. Additional garnishes can include lime wedges, cilantro, coconut flakes or chutney.

Mung Soup with Greens

30 – 35 minutes
Yields about 3 – 4 servings

1 tsp mustard seeds

2 tsp cumin seeds

4 – 6 curry leaves

2 Tbsp fresh ginger, finely grated

¼ tsp turmeric powder

Pinch of asafoetida powder/hing

1 cup yellow split mung dal

1 medium zucchini, diced small

Two handfuls of greens, finely chopped (spinach, kale, chard)

Sea salt to taste

½ cup cilantro leaves

Juice of ½ lemon

1. In a large pot, dry roast mustard and cumin seeds over medium heat until they begin to pop. Add mung dal and remaining spices and pour 4 cups of boiling water over top. Lower heat, cover and simmer about 20 minutes, stirring occasionally.
2. When mung begins to get soft, add zucchini and replace lid. Cook another 5 minutes.
3. Add greens and sea salt, stir and cook another 5 minutes.
4. Add cilantro leaves and lemon juice, stir just to combine, and ladle soup into bowls. Serve hot.

Thyme for a Change Mung Soup

30 – 35 minutes
Yields about 3 – 4 servings

1 cup mung dal

3 cups water

1 tsp sea salt

1 – 2 stalks celery, chopped

1 tsp dried thyme

Pinch hing or asafeotida

Juice of ½ lemon, or more to taste

Handful chopped parsley for garnish

1. Place all ingredients except lemon juice and parsley in a medium pot.
2. Bring to a boil over medium-high heat, lower heat to simmer and cook, stirring often, until all the water is absorbed, about 20 minutes.
3. Stir in lemon juice and serve hot.

Mung Bean Burgers

½ cup mung beans, soaked and drained

1 tsp cumin

½ tsp salt

1 tsp fresh thyme

1 tsp fresh dill

¼ tsp paprika

1 egg

¼ cup quick oat flakes or ½ cup cooked rice

1 leek, chopped

Fresh basil (optional)

20 minutes, plus 2 hours soaking time
Yields about 8 patties

1. Soak the mung beans for at least 2 hours, drain and combine in food processor with cumin, salt and fresh herbs. Grind until a sticky, uniform texture is achieved.
2. Place ground mung and spices in bowl and add egg, oats and chopped leek. Stir well.
3. Heat a skillet with ghee and form mixture into patties. Cook on medium heat, each side about 4-5 minutes. Alternately, you can lightly grease a cookie sheet and bake burgers. Serve with Parsley Sauce (page 189) and/or a chutney (pages 183 - 184).

Variation:
When not cleansing, try adding 4 oz of feta cheese when adding egg, oats and leek.

Rejuvenation Phase Recipes

Ginger Lemon Appetizer

5 minutes
Yields about 20 servings

3 inch hunk of fresh ginger root

Lemon or lime

Sea salt

1. Peel ginger and cut into thin slices. Lay out in a single layer on a cutting board or plate.
2. Squeeze lemon or lime juice over slices and sprinkle with sea salt.
3. Place slices in an airtight container and store in the refrigerator. Eat one or two slices 10 - 15 minutes before meals to stimulate digestion.

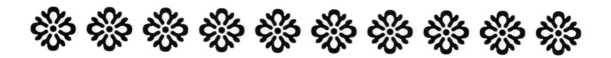

Probiotic Almond Cheese Spread

15 minutes, plus fermentation
Yields about 1 cup

1 cup raw almonds, soaked overnight and drained

½ tsp sea salt, or to taste

¼ cup water

A few Tbsp sauerkraut brine or probiotic powder (open and empty about 1 or 2 capsules)

Minced fresh herbs, such as rosemary and thyme (optional)

1 – 4 cloves garlic, minced or grated (optional)

1. Blanch soaked almonds by covering them in boiling water and let sit a few minutes. Drain and slip the skins off.
2. Combine water, sea salt and peeled almonds in a food processor and blend until smooth, stopping to scrape down the sides of the bowl. Add more water if needed to get a thick, spreadable texture.
3. Add brine or probiotic powder and mix well.
4. Pour blended almonds into a large jar and cover the top with a piece of cloth or plastic wrap, securing it with a rubber band. Store in a cool, dark place overnight or until the desired sourness is achieved; taste every 12 hours. (This may take up to 3 days in cooler climates.) The cheese will bubble up during this fermentation process.
5. Add herbs and garlic, if using, and stir well.
6. Store in an airtight glass container in the refrigerator until ready to serve. Try with the Rosemary Crackers on the next page.

Rosemary Crackers

20 minutes
Yields about 20 crackers

1½ cups almond flour

1 Tbsp sesame seeds

1 Tbsp flax seeds

½ tsp sea salt

1 tsp rosemary, minced

3 – 4 dried figs, chopped

1 large egg, beaten

1 Tbsp olive oil

1. In a large mixing bowl, stir together almond flour, seeds, salt, rosemary and figs.
2. Mix in egg and oil until well combined.
3. Roll out dough between 2 sheets of parchment paper until ⅛ inch thick. Cut into 2 inch squares using a knife or pizza cutter.
4. Bake at 350° for 10-12 minutes until golden brown. Cool and serve.

Rice & Red Lentil Dosa

30 minutes, plus soaking & fermentation time
Yields about ten 8" dosai

A dosa is a traditional Indian fermented pancake that is very thin, similar to a crepe. Any number of fillings can be enjoyed with these.

1 cup white basmati rice (or other non-sticky white rice)

½ cup red lentils

2 tsp sea salt

Optional:
1 tsp grated fresh ginger

½ tsp ground cumin

½ tsp ground coriander

2 gloves garlic, grated or minced

⅛ cup finely minced onion

1. Rinse rice and lentils and sort through to pick out any pebbles or other foreign material. In a large bowl, cover with warm water, then cover bowl with a damp towel. Allow to sit overnight, or about 8 hours.
2. Drain off water and grind in a food processor on high for about 3 - 5 minutes, until a thick, even consistency is reached, adding water as needed. A fairly thin pancake-like batter is desired. The better the mixture is ground, the better the dosai will turn out.
3. Place mixture in a bowl and cover with a damp towel again and allow to ferment, about 12 - 48 hours.
4. Add optional ingredients and stir to combine. Heat a skillet over medium heat and warm a teaspoon of oil, ghee or butter. Cook like pancakes, several minutes on each side. Enjoy alone or fill with vegetables, potatoes or yogurt.

Coconut Rice

25 – 35 minutes
Yields about 3 – 6 servings

2 cups white or brown basmati rice

1 can (14 oz.) coconut milk

1 ¾ cups water

4 lemongrass stalks, bottoms and outer stalks removed

2 cloves garlic, grated or minced

2 Tbsp grated fresh ginger

½ cup shredded unsweetened coconut

2 tsp sea salt, or to taste

1 cup thinly sliced green onions

½ cup fresh cilantro, chopped

1. Crush lemongrass by pounding it with a wooden spoon.
2. Place all ingredients except green onion and cilantro in a large pot and bring to a boil. Lower heat to simmer and cook until all liquid is absorbed, about 15 - 20 minutes for white rice or 25- 35 minutes for brown rice.
3. Allow to cool slightly, remove lemongrass stalks and add green onion and cilantro. Garnish with additional shredded coconut and serve.

Variation:
This recipe is still delicious without the lemongrass, so if you don't have it on hand, make this anyway.

Thai Coconut Shrimp Soup

20 minutes
Yields about 4 servings

2 cups canned coconut milk

*2 cups chicken or vegetable stock or water
(pages 198 - 199)*

½ - 1 lb. shrimp (raw & shelled)

*2 stalks lemongrass, cut into 2" long
pieces and crushed*

12 slices dried galangal root (or 6 fresh)

*3 fresh kaffir lime leaves or 6 dried
leaves, torn into small pieces*

2 cloves garlic, chopped

1 tsp sea salt

¼ tsp freshly ground black pepper

1 medium carrot, sliced into matchsticks

3 Tbsp fresh lime juice

2 green onions, thinly sliced

Handful fresh cilantro, finely chopped

1 - 2 cups cooked rice

1. Place coconut milk, broth or water, lemongrass, galangal root, kaffir lime leaves, garlic, salt and black pepper in a large pot or wok and bring to a boil over medium heat.
2. Add carrot and cook 5 minutes.
3. Add shrimp and cook another 3 to 5 minutes, until shrimp turns pink. Stir often.
4. Just before serving, add lime juice, green onion and fresh cilantro and stir.
5. Place a scoop of cooked rice in the bottom of each bowl and ladle hot soup over top. Garnish with additional cilantro and serve hot.

Note:
Galangal root is also known as Thai ginger and can usually be found in its dried form in most health food stores. If you can't find it, substitute 1" sliced fresh ginger root.

Spinach Paneer

20 minutes
Yields about 2 – 4 servings

2 Tbsp coconut oil

3 cloves garlic, grated or minced

1 tsp turmeric

1 ½ tsp cumin

1 tsp coriander

¼ tsp cloves

¼ tsp cayenne (omit for pitta)

1 tsp salt

5-7 crimini mushrooms, sliced

1 cup chopped green beans

1- 2 bunches spinach

4 oz. paneer cheese, cut into cubes

Handful of fresh cilantro, chopped, for garnish

Lime wedges for garnish

1. Sauté garlic in coconut oil until it just begins to turn golden, then add the rest of the spices.
2. Add green beans and mushrooms to pan and coat with spices. Sauté another 5-7 minutes.
3. Add spinach and paneer and cook for 5 more minutes, covered, over low heat.
4. Garnish with chopped cilantro and lime. Serve with brown rice or other grain and a side of chutney.

Nourishing Cookies

30 minutes
Yields about 12 cookies

1 ½ cups whole raw almonds

6 - 7 large Medjool dates, pitted and roughly chopped

2 Tbsp coconut oil

¼ tsp cardamom

½ tsp cinnamon

1 Tbsp vanilla

¼ tsp salt

1. Preheat oven to 350° and grease a baking sheet with ghee or coconut oil.
2. Place almonds in a food processor and pulse for several minutes until coarsely chopped.
3. Add remaining ingredients and pulse again until a thick, sticky dough is created.
4. Form dough into 2 inch diameter balls, place on greased baking sheet and flatten a bit. (You can also form a well in the center to be filled with jam after baking, if desired.)
5. Bake for approximately 12-15 minutes or until lightly brown. Allow to cool slightly (they will crumble a bit if eaten directly from the oven) and enjoy.

Simple Date Squares

20 minutes, plus 2 hours refrigeration
Yields about 16 squares

Crust Ingredients:

2 cups blanched almond flour

8 pitted dates, soaked and drained

¼ cup coconut oil

½ tsp sea salt

Filling Ingredients:

2 cups pitted dates, soaked and drained, ¼ cup soaking water reserved

½ tsp vanilla extract

¼ tsp sea salt

¼ tsp ground cardamom

⅛ tsp ground nutmeg

1. Line an 8" x 8" baking dish with parchment paper.
2. In a food processor, combine crust ingredients and process until a sticky dough is formed. Set aside 1 cup of this for the crumble topping and press the rest into the bottom of the prepared baking dish. Use your hands to press it evenly.
3. Combine the filling ingredients, including the reserved soaking water in the food processor and process until a thick paste is created. Spread this filling over the crust, then sprinkle the remaining almond meal mixture on top. Press topping gently into the date filling.
4. Refrigerate 2 hours, or until set firm. Cut into 2" squares and serve chilled for best texture. Store in an airtight container for up to 7 days.

Fruit Compote

30 minutes
Yields about 3 cups

1 cup orange juice

1 cinnamon stick

½ tsp anise seeds

½ tsp grated lemon rind

1 tsp grated orange rind

1 lb peach slices, fresh or frozen and
thawed

1 lb. pitted cherries, fresh or frozen
and thawed

2 navel oranges, sliced and peeled

¼ cup raw honey

⅓ cup toasted seeds

1. Combine orange juice, spices, and rinds
   in a medium pot. Bring to a boil, reduce
   heat, and cook uncovered about 5 minutes.
   Strain out seeds and rinds, then add fruit
   to the spiced juice.
2. Return mixture to the cooking pot and
   bring to a boil. Lower heat and simmer 15
   minutes.
3. Remove from heat, cool a little* and add
   honey. Serve warm or at room temperature, topped with seeds.

Note: Honey becomes toxic when heated,
causing ama and blockage of the channels.
When using honey as a sweetener, make sure
the food or drink is cool enough to insert a
pinky into without getting burned.

Slow Rice Pudding

2 hours 20 minutes
Yields about 6 servings

1 cup cooked white or brown rice

3 ½ cups unsweetened soy or almond milk

Finely grated rind of 1 lemon

1 tsp ground nutmeg

½ tsp ground cinnamon

Pinch of ground cloves

½ cup organic raisins or chopped dates

2 eggs, separated

⅔ cup canned coconut milk

1 ½ tsp pure vanilla extract

Pinch of sea salt

1. Preheat oven to 300° and oil a deep pie dish.
2. In a medium pot, combine rice, milk, ½ tsp nutmeg, cinnamon, cloves and raisins or dates and simmer for 15-20 minutes until very thick, stirring often.
3. Remove from heat and allow to cool slightly. Add egg yolks, coconut milk, vanilla and salt. Stir well.
4. Beat egg whites until fluffy and fold into the rice mixture.
5. Pour into oiled pie dish, top with remaining nutmeg and bake approximately 2 hours, until the center is cooked through and the top begins to brown. Enjoy warm or hot, topped with a little ghee.

Variation:
For a quick version, simply follow steps one and two, add coconut milk, vanilla and sea salt and enjoy!

Nutty Flourless Granola Bars

30 minutes
Yields about 20 squares

8 large dates, pitted and chopped

¼ cup coconut oil

¼ cup hazelnut, hemp or almond milk

1 Tbsp vanilla

1 Tbsp chia seeds

1 ½ cups oats

¼ cup chopped cashews

¼ cup chopped almonds

1 - 2 Tbsp maple syrup

¼ cup hemp seeds

½ tsp sea salt

¾ tsp baking soda

¼ cup cacao nibs

1. Preheat oven to 350° and grease a baking sheet with ghee or coconut oil.
2. Put dates, coconut oil, nut milk, vanilla and chia seeds in a food processor and pulse until a thick paste is formed.
3. In a large bowl, combine oats, chopped nuts, seeds, syrup, salt and baking soda. Stir in paste, then add cacao nibs and stir again until everything is evenly distributed.
4. Lay out a large sheet of parchment paper (approximately 9" x 11") on a cutting board or counter. Press mixture into a large rectangle and cut into 2" squares. Arrange on the prepared baking sheet. Bake for 12-15 minutes.

Banana Almond Meal Protein Muffins

60 minutes
Yields 12 muffins

2 ½ cups blanched almond flour
(or 1 ½ cups almond flour and 1 cup
brown rice flour)

1 Tbsp cinnamon

2 tsp baking soda

1 tsp sea salt

2 carrots, finely grated

1 large apple, peeled and finely grated

½ cup unsweetened shredded coconut

½ cup raisins or other dried fruit

½ cup chopped dates

3 eggs, beaten

1 ripe banana, mashed

½ cup coconut oil

1. Preheat oven to 350° and line or oil a muffin tin.
2. In a large bowl, combine everything except the eggs, banana and coconut oil and stir to combine.
3. In a smaller bowl combine remaining wet ingredients and beat well.
4. Pour wet ingredients into dry ingredients and stir to combine.
5. Pour batter equally into 12 muffins cups and bake 30-40 minutes, or until a fork inserted into the center comes out clean. Store these in an airtight container in the fridge.

Blissful Goji Date Balls

10 minutes
Yields about 12 balls

3 Tbsp coconut oil

½ cup shredded unsweetened coconut

½ cup raw almonds

6 - 8 large dates, pitted and chopped

¼ cup goji berries

¼ cup carob or cocoa powder

1 Tbsp maple syrup (optional)

Pinch of sea salt

1. Place all ingredients in the work bowl of a food processor.
2. Process until a sticky, even mixture is formed.
3. Roll into balls and enjoy!

Lemon Ginger Macaroons

40 minutes
Yields about 24 macaroons

2 cups finely shredded unsweetened coconut

½ cup blanched almond flour

½ cup maple syrup

2 eggs, beaten

2 inch hunk of ginger, peeled and grated

Zest of 1 lemon

2 tsp vanilla

1. Preheat oven to 350° and line a baking sheet with parchment paper.
2. Combine all ingredients in a bowl and mix well. Let sit for 10 minutes to allow moisture to be absorbed.
3. Scoop out 1 Tbsp of mixture at a time, place on parchment-lined baking sheet and flatten out a bit.
4. Bake 15-20 minutes or until golden. Allow to cool and set for 20 minutes before removing.

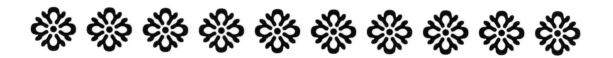

Coconut Buckwheat Granola

30 minutes
Yields about 3 cups

1 cup quinoa flakes

½ cup buckwheat groats (sometimes called kasha)

½ cup chopped or slivered almonds

¼ cup flax seeds

¼ cup pumpkin seeds

¼ cup coconut oil, melted

¼ cup maple syrup

2 Tbsp ground cinnamon

½ tsp sea salt, or to taste

½ cup shredded, unsweetened coconut

¼ cup raisins or currants

1. Preheat oven to 300° and line a baking sheet with parchment.
2. In a large bowl, combine all ingredients except shredded coconut and raisins. Stir to coat.
3. Spread onto lined baking sheet and bake 10 minutes.
4. Remove from oven, add coconut, stir and bake another 8 minutes.
5. Cool completely, add raisins, and store in an airtight container.

Guilt-Free Fudge Balls

10 minutes
Yields about 18 balls

6 - 7 large dates, preferably Medjool, chopped

1 cup walnuts

3 Tbsp cocoa or carob powder

1 tsp vanilla extract

⅛ tsp sea salt

1. Place all ingredients in the work bowl of a food processor.
2. Pulse on high until smooth.
3. Remove from food processor and roll into little balls. Serve immediately or store in an airtight container in the refrigerator. (You might want to double the recipe, in case the first batch is gone by the time you are finished rolling into balls.)

Variation:
Try adding ¼ cup of any of your favorite dried fruits, such as goji berries or cherries.

Maple Sesame Bon Bons

1 Tbsp sesame seeds, ground

2 Tbsp almond butter

½ inch fresh ginger, grated

2 tsp maple syrup

⅛ tsp cardamom

¼ tsp cinnamon

2 Tbsp finely shredded unsweetened coconut

1. In a medium bowl, combine all ingredients except coconut. Stir until everything is evenly distributed.
2. Form mixture into 6 balls, then roll in coconut. Serve immediately or store in an airtight container on the counter or in the refrigerator.

Rasayana Drink

*1 cup almond milk or raw
non-homogenized milk*

*A dash of each cardamom, nutmeg and
cinnamon*

½ tsp vanilla

1 - 2 dates

5 -7 raw almonds

1 tsp ghee or coconut oil

1. In a small pot, warm milk and spices.
2. Place the warm milk, vanilla, dates and
   almonds in a blender or food processor
   and blend until smooth.
3. Pour into a glass and add ghee or oil.
   Drink warm before bed.

Bibliography

Atreya (2001). Perfect balance. New York, Penguin Putnam.

Boccio, Frank Jude (2004). Mindfulness Yoga. Somerville: Wisdom Publications.

Daniluk, Julie (2011). Meals that heal inflammation. New York: Hay House.

Douillard, Dr. John (2011). The colorado cleanse. Boulder: LifeSpa Products, LLC.

Fife, Bruce, M.D. "Coconut oil as treatment for alcoholism." *Well Being Jounral.* v. 22, n. 6, p9-14. Print.

Frawley, Dr. David (2000). Ayurvedic healing. Twin Lakes: Lotus Press.

Frawley, Dr. David (1999). Yoga and ayurveda. Twin Lakes: Lotus Press.

Frawley, Dr. David (1996). Ayurveda and the mind. Twin Lakes: Lotus Press.

Gates, Donna (2011). The body ecology diet. New York: Hay House.

Haas, Elson M., MD (2012). The detox diet. New York: Ten Speed Press.

Herron, Robert E., John B. Fagan. "Lipophil-mediated reduction of toxicants in humans: an evaluation of an ayurvedic detoxification procedure." *Alternative Therapies.* Sept/Oct 2002. v. 8 n. 5. p40-51. Print

Johnson RJ and Gower T. (2009). The sugar fix: the high-fructose fallout that is making you sick and fat. Gallery Books.

Joshi, Sunil V. M.D.(Ayu) (1996). Ayurveda and panchakarma.Wisconsin: Lotus Press.

Katz, Rebecca with Mat Edelson (2013). The longevity kitchen. New York: Ten Speed Press.

Krishan, Shubhra (2003). The essential ayurveda. Novato: New World Library.

Bibliography

Lad, Vasant B.A.M.S., M.A.Sc. (2002). Textbook of ayurveda: fundamental principles. Albuquerque: The Ayurvedic Press.

Lad, Vasant B.A.M.S., M.A.Sc. (1998) The complete book of ayurvedic home remedies. New York: Three Rivers Press.

Lutzker, Talya (2012). The ayurvedic vegan kitchen. Summertown: Book Publishing Company.

Martin, Jeanne Marie (2000). Complete candida yeast guidebook. Roseville: Prima Publishing.

Robertson, Laurel (1976). Laurel's kitchen. Petaluma: Nilgiri Press.

Thomas, Anna (1972). The vegetarian epicure. New York: Vintage Books.

Pole, Sebastian (2006). Ayurvedic medicine. Philadelphia: Elsevier Limited.

Svoboda, Dr. Robert E. (1998) Prakriti. Twin Lakes: Lotus Press.

Svoboda, Dr. Robert E. (1999) Ayurveda for Women. United Kingdom: David & Charles.

Yarema, Thomas, M.D. with Daniel Rhoda and Johnny Brannigan (2006). Eat taste heal. Kapaa: Five Elements Press.

Index

About the Authors

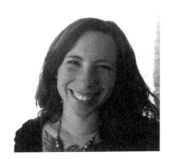

Adrian Nowland

Adrian Nowland is an Ayurvedic Wellness Counselor and Holistic Health Coach. She is board certified by the American Association of Drugless Practitioners and is a member of the National Ayurvedic Medical Association. She studied at Kerala Ayurveda Academy and the Institute for Integrative Nutrition, as well as attending various Ayurvedic workshops and classes. She leads group programs, retreats and workshops that share the wisdom of Ayurveda so that others may benefit from the rich teachings. For more information on her offerings, please go to laughingblossom.com. At the time of this writing, Adrian lives in sunny North Central Washington with her husband and their spunky daughter.

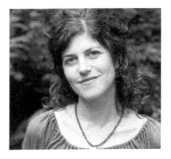

Ronly Blau

Ronly Blau is a Certified Ayurvedic Practitioner and Yoga Teacher. She studied Ayurveda at the Mount Madonna Institute and in Kerala, India. She offers Ayurvedic health consultations and has been leading cleanse groups since 2008. A yoga teacher since 2000, she studied with Kathleen Hunt, and completed the Mindfulness Yoga & Meditation Training at Spirit Rock Meditation Center. She is informed by her longtime practice in Yoga and vipassana meditation and enjoys holding a space for healing, learning and spiritual growth. Ronly leads classes, workshops and retreats in both Ayurveda and Yoga. Please visit her website: www.MeadowHeartAyurveda.com for more information on her offerings. She makes her home on Vashon Island with her husband and two daughters.

CPSIA information can be obtained
at www.ICGtesting.com
Printed in the USA
BVHW05s0351070418
512695BV00006B/124/P

9 780692 646779